Women's Sexual Health and Dysfunction - Clinical Practice, Integrative Therapies, and Contemporary Challenges

Edited by Dhastagir Sultan Sheriff, Abubakr Nasr and Öznur Dündar Akın

Published in London, United Kingdom

Women's Sexual Health and Dysfunction - Clinical Practice, Integrative Therapies, and Contemporary Challenges
http://dx.doi.org/10.5772/intechopen.1010367
Edited by Dhastagir Sultan Sheriff, Abubakr Nasr and Öznur Dündar Akın

Contributors
Ana Claudia F. Amaral, Andrea Patricia Chancay Mendoza, Ava G. Grotting, César Oswaldo Loor Loor, Deborah Denisse Gaibor Santos, Dhastagir Sultan Sheriff, Diaa-Eldin Taha, Diogo A. Folly, Débora de Castro Soares, Elaine Cristina Ferreira Dias, Elizabeth C. Bottorff, Fabiene Bernardes Castro Vale, Gabriel León San Miguel, Ibrahim Alowidah, Jefferson R. A. Silva, Juan Carlos Suárez Fernández, Karishma Hemmady, Laura de Siqueira Khouri, Liliana Carolina Torres Vélez, Manopriya Thiruvagounder, María Fernanda Calderón León, Mohamed Tharwat, Perianayagi Palavesam, Ramona Ramasamy, Reham Ramadan, Rogger Isaac Chinga Acuña, Shankar Shanmugam Rajendran, Sonnia Paola Diaz Cepeda, Srinidhi Satish, Viviana Carolina Torres Vélez, Yusuf Ziya Kizildemir

First published in London, United Kingdom, 2026 by IntechOpen
IntechOpen is the global imprint of INTECHOPEN LIMITED, registered in England and Wales, registration number: 11086078, 167-169 Great Portland Street, London, W1W 5PF, United Kingdom

For EU product safety concerns: IN TECH d.o.o., Prolaz Marije Krucifikse Kozulić 3, 51000 Rijeka, Croatia, info@intechopen.com or visit our website at intechopen.com.

British Library Cataloguing-in-Publication Data
A catalogue record for this book is available from the British Library

Women's Sexual Health and Dysfunction - Clinical Practice, Integrative Therapies, and Contemporary Challenges
Edited by Dhastagir Sultan Sheriff, Abubakr Nasr and Öznur Dündar Akın
p. cm.

This title is part of the Obstetrics and Gynecology Book Series, Volume 14
Topic: Reproductive and Gynecologic Health
Series Editor: Zouhair O. Amarin
Topic Editor: Courtney Marsh

Print ISBN 978-1-80631-046-3
Online ISBN 978-1-80631-045-6
eBook (PDF) ISBN 978-1-80631-047-0
ISSN 3049-706X

IntechOpen Book Series

Obstetrics and Gynecology

Volume 14

Aims and Scope of the Series

Obstetrics and Gynecology field typically covers several subspecialties that include maternal-fetal medicine, gynecologic oncology, reproductive endocrinology and subfertility, urogynecology and female pelvic reconstructive surgery, critical care medicine, complex family planning, pediatric and adolescent gynecology, menopausal and geriatric gynecology, and minimally invasive gynecologic surgery.
Apart from being diverse, obstetrics and gynecology is a challenging and demanding specialty. It combines medical and surgical skills.
The sequence of books in this series will have certain characteristics in common that will be recognized as part of the same informative multi-volume book programme.

Meet the Series Editor

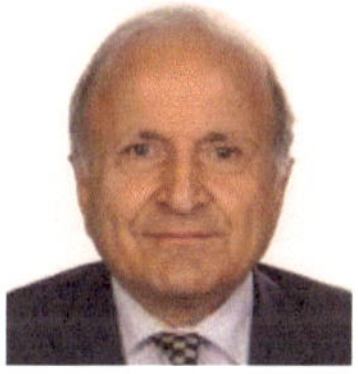

Zouhair Amarin is a Professor of Obstetrics and Gynaecology at the Jordan University of Science and Technology. He was previously a lecturer at the University of Glasgow, Scotland, a senior lecturer at the University of Nottingham, England, and the dean of the Faculty of Medicine at Mutah University, Jordan. Professor Amarin is a fellow of the Royal College of Obstetricians and Gynaecologists, and the Faculty of Public Health, London. He holds master's degrees in medical science and medical education. He is a pioneer in IVF and was the first in the world to develop microsurgical epididymis sperm aspiration for clinical use. He also discovered a surgical procedure for critical ovarian hyperstimulation syndrome. Professor Amarin has edited books, authored book chapters, and published more than 130 papers. He is the recipient of eight awards.

Meet the Volume Editors

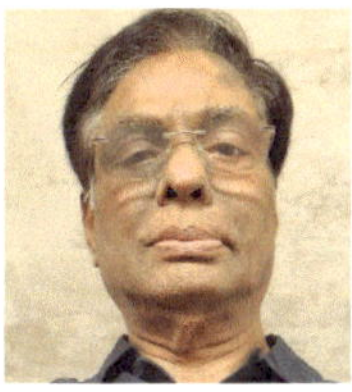

Dhastagir Sultan Sheriff is a member of the European Society for Human Reproduction and Early Human Development, the Association of Physiologists and Pharmacologists of India, and the National Academy of Medical Sciences, New Delhi. He is also a resource person for UNESCO. Dr. Sheriff has authored five books, including a textbook on medical biochemistry, and has additional interests in human sexology. He has published editorials in the British Journal of Sexology, Journal of the Royal Society of Medicine, Postgraduate Medicine, and The Scientist. He was a former Rotarian, Citizen Ambassador, and was selected for the Ford Foundation Fellowship.

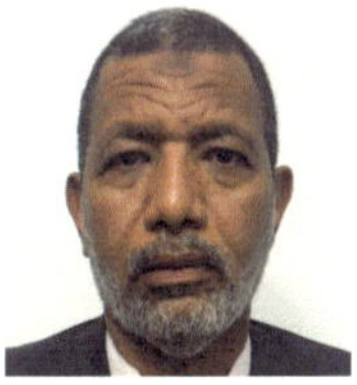

Abubakr Nasr is an Associate Professor at the Faculty of Medicine, University of Khartoum, and is currently a senior consultant at the National Guard Hospital in Madina. Dr. Nasr has long academic experience as a medical teacher and trainer. Research and publications included 28 publications, including two chapters on ovarian cancer screening and uterine incision, as shown in the ResearchGate profile (https://www. researchgate. net/profile/Abubakr-Nasr?ev=hdr_xprf). Dr. Nasr has extensive clinical expertise in gynecologic disorders affecting women's health across the lifespan, including female sexual dysfunction, pelvic pathology, and complex cesarean delivery.

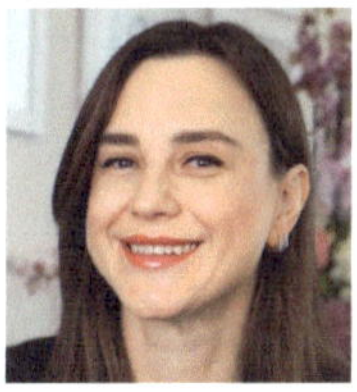

Dr. Öznur Dündar Akın is an Assistant Professor (Doktor Öğretim Üyesi) in the Department of Obstetrics and Gynecology at Atlas University, Istanbul. She earned her Medical Degree from Istanbul University Cerrahpaşa Faculty of Medicine in 2007 and completed her residency in 2013. She also holds an MBA from Istanbul Aydın University. Dr. Akın maintains a dual career in academia and clinical practice; alongside her faculty position at Atlas University, she provides expert care at her private clinical practice in Istanbul. Her clinical expertise is supported by specialized training in Sexual Dysfunction, Urodynamics, and Genital Esthetics. She has published numerous articles in high-impact international journals and continues to contribute to the field through both her academic research and clinical experience, focusing on integrative and contemporary approaches to women's health.

Contents

Preface

Female sexual dysfunction (FSD) has become a major issue in female sexual health. While sexual health provides a holistic approach to tackling sexual problems, including FSD, female sexuality remains a taboo in many societies. Male dominance and female hesitancy often hinder open discussions; consequently, female sexual dysfunction is frequently diagnosed accidentally when couples seek help for infertility.

Infertility clinics rely predominantly on genetic and laboratory testing, a fragmented approach that may be attributed to cultural diversity and the social determinants of public health. This fragmentation is evident in how human sexuality and infertility are handled; for instance, conditions like male infertility may be noted for their multiple effects on physical health without giving due prominence to the associated sexual dysfunction.

The present monograph on female sexual dysfunction provides a mosaic of interrelated issues in female sexual health and sexuality across eight chapters.

1. Interconnected Challenges in Female Sexual Dysfunction: Clinical Access, Regulatory Policy, and Research Challenges to Novel Treatments

2. Misinformation on Digital Platforms about the Use of Medicinal Plants and Herbal Medicines: The Search for Managing Climacteric Symptoms

3. Female Sexual Dysfunction and Urinary Incontinence

4. Sexual Dysfunction in Polycystic Ovary Syndrome (PCOS): A Biopsychosocial Approach to Assessment and Management

5. Polycystic Ovary Syndrome: A Therapeutic Challenge

6. Management of Hypoactive Sexual Desire Disorder

7. Sexual Dysfunction Among Women with Type 2 Diabetes Mellitus

8. Lichen Sclerosus and Its Impact on Female Sexual Dysfunction: A Comprehensive Review

Key highlights include the exploration of female dysfunction alongside interconnected challenges in clinical access, regulation, and novel treatments.

These disorders are to be diagnosed only when they cause significant distress, and not when they are merely a consequence of inadequate sexual stimulation or relationship factors.

Dr. Dhastagir Sultan Sheriff
Anna Medical College,
Montagne Blanche, Mauritius

American University of Sovereign Nations (AUSN),
Los Angeles, USA

Associate Prof. Abubakr Nasr
University of Khartoum,
Khartoum, Sudan

Dr. Öznur Dündar Akın
Atlas Üniversitesi,
Istanbul, Türkiye

Chapter 1

Interconnected Challenges in Female Sexual Dysfunction: Clinical Access, Regulatory Policy, and Research Challenges to Novel Treatments

Elizabeth C. Bottorff, Ava G. Grotting and Srinidhi Satish

Abstract

Female sexual dysfunction (FSD) affects up to 40% of women worldwide, yet treatment options remain severely limited compared to male sexual dysfunction therapies. While many authors have discussed the complex biopsychosocial interactions that complicate FSD diagnosis and treatment, the infrastructural barriers within which scientists and clinicians operate are often overlooked. This chapter examines how clinical, regulatory, and scientific perspectives create an interconnected web of challenges that impede novel FSD treatment development. Clinical barriers form the most immediate obstacles patients encounter. Healthcare providers lack specialized training in sexual medicine, with medical schools providing inadequate education. Both patients and providers face unique challenges navigating sexual health discussions, compounded by stigma and cultural barriers that limit treatment accessibility. Regulatory perspectives reveal additional systemic problems. Diagnostic inconsistencies between DSM-5 classifications and professional society recommendations create confusion in treatment targets. Even when properly diagnosed, insurance coverage gaps persist, as sexual health is often categorized as a quality-of-life issue rather than a medical necessity. Furthermore, few FDA-approved treatments exist for women compared to male sexual dysfunction. Scientific barriers underpin these downstream challenges. FDA approval requires preclinical and clinical testing, yet animal models translate poorly to complex female sexual responses. Clinical testing faces extraordinary challenges, including difficulty establishing clinically meaningful endpoints given multifaceted biopsychosocial interactions, recruitment difficulties with self-selection bias, and unrealistic laboratory conditions. Research infrastructure remains compromised by historical male-dominated perspectives and persistent funding disparities. This chapter illustrates how these interconnected barriers perpetuate the treatment gap and concludes with potential solutions for systemic change.

Keywords: translational research, study design, research infrastructure, insurance coverage, FDA regulatory pathway, access to care, patient-reported outcomes

1. Introduction

Female sexual dysfunction (FSD) is highly prevalent yet remains underdiagnosed, undertreated, and under-researched. Barriers to care arise at every stage of the clinical and research pipeline. At the patient level, sociocultural stigma, limited access to specialized clinics, and inadequate provider training restrict entry into care. Within the healthcare system, diagnostic ambiguity and inconsistent treatment frameworks hinder accurate classification and management, while reimbursement policies and regulatory processes create additional obstacles to accessing therapy. Finally, in research settings, methodological challenges, ranging from outcome selection to trial design, constrain the development of new interventions. This chapter traces these barriers sequentially, beginning with obstacles in the clinical setting, then examining regulatory and policy hurdles, and concluding with scientific limitations that slow therapeutic innovation.

2. Healthcare system and clinical access barriers

Women seeking care for FSD face structural, sociocultural, and educational barriers at every step, from limited specialized services and inconsistent guidelines to stigma and lack of awareness. Providers often encounter gaps in training and resources, creating a system where diagnosis and treatment are uneven and frequently delayed. The following sections examine how healthcare infrastructure, patient factors, and provider preparedness shape access and outcomes in FSD care.

2.1 Healthcare system structure

Women seeking care for FSD face many barriers within the healthcare system at each step of receiving comprehensive care. There are many barriers, including a profound lack of specialized sexual health services and limited provider training or standardized guidelines. Patient-related factors, such as stigma, embarrassment, and limited awareness of available interventions, further compound these challenges.

Patients' access to specialized health services is limited by geography and the scope of available sexual health services. One study found that seven states lack any clinics providing FSD services, and 26 states do not have any clinics specializing in female sexual health [1]. Of the clinics the study did identify, only 17% of sexual medicine clinics were affiliated with academic institutions, reflecting the broader lack of exposure to female sexual medicine in the environments where providers receive training. Many of the clinics identified as specializing in female sexual medicine are private, offering investigational therapies of unclear efficacy, often operated by providers without formal training in sexual medicine. Additionally, 23% of these clinics were identified as primarily focusing on esthetics and elective procedures, which are unlikely to be covered by insurance. Inconsistencies in the availability and delivery of FSD care place an added burden on patients, who must locate providers or clinics capable of meeting their needs. For those without local options, financial constraints or insurance limitations may prevent them from seeking care elsewhere. Additionally, the use of investigational treatments could pose challenges for patients who need to use insurance to afford the cost of medical care.

While there are some standardized recommendations for the care of FSD patients, management of female sexual function is not routinely practiced in a primary care context [2]. Clinical recommendations for the treatment of FSD encompass a complex assessment of the biopsychosocial factors that affect sexual function, including patient interviews, laboratory investigations, physical examinations, and self-report questionnaires [3]. When patients present to primary care with concerns about their sexual health, their providers are often unable to provide adequate management. This gap in care is highlighted when compared to men's sexual health. For example, one study found that when women with FSD are diagnosed by primary care providers, they are significantly less likely to receive care that is appropriately aligned with the current literature [2]. FSD patients in these primary care settings also have a lower likelihood of receiving appropriate management of their condition, with the median management rate at around 25% compared to 52% management for male patients with erectile dysfunction (ED).

Because many cases of FSD go undiagnosed in primary care, most patients are managed by gynecologists. However, only about 2.4% of women with FSD receive a formal referral to see a specialist in Obstetrics and Gynecology (OB/GYN) [2]. In a survey of primary care physicians, 90% reported little confidence in diagnosing hypoactive sexual desire disorder (HSDD). Additionally, 90% had never screened for it, and 98% had never prescribed medication for it [4]. This likely reflects inadequate training and familiarity with FSD in both primary care and specialty care, as well as limited knowledge of current and emerging treatment options [5]. Together, these findings reflect inadequate training and awareness in both primary and specialty care, which limits referrals and perpetuates disparities in how male and FSDs are managed.

2.2 Patient related factors

The structural and sociocultural frameworks surrounding sexual healthcare contribute to barriers for both patients and providers when initiating discussions about FSD. For patients, contextual factors such as relationship dynamics, life stressors, religious or cultural messaging around sexuality, and barriers to health literacy may affect their comfort in discussing their sexual health in a medical setting [5]. While many states mandate sexual health education in United States public schools, only 38% of states require this education to be medically accurate, and actual content varies by state and region [6]. One study found that 74% of sex education teachers use abstinence-only education, but only 33% supplemented this content with curricula that cover other areas of sexual health [7]. This education framework could contribute to less access to comprehensive sexual health knowledge that may help people identify sexual function concerns. An additional preclinical factor affecting taboos could include religious views regarding sexual health. One study found that religious service participation among women is correlated with less sexual health service utilization [8]. Beyond this, several factors contribute to patients feeling hesitant to seek care for FSD in a clinical setting.

A web-based survey questioned 3,807 healthy women about their experiences seeking help from a physician regarding their sexual health concerns [9].

Forty percent of respondents reported not seeking medical advice; of these, 54% indicated that they wanted to seek care. Their reasons for not seeking care included embarrassment, the belief that the physician wouldn't be able to help, or not recognizing sexual health as an appropriate topic for medical consultation. Many patients avoid or fear bringing up sexual health topics in a clinical encounter due to the reactions of their providers. The responses identified in the survey included embarrassed silences, expressions of surprise, provision of misinformation, inattentiveness, belittlement, or advice shaped by the physician's personal values. Such responses may feel invalidating; only 39% of patients in the survey believed their provider understood the significance of their concern, and only 26% were thoroughly examined [9].

Patients' perceptions of provider discomfort are corroborated by physicians' self-reports. Providers may feel unequipped to assess concerns related to FSD. A qualitative study of primary care physicians experienced in treating FSD described physicians as hesitant to discuss concerns that they feel unable to treat effectively [10]. As a result, these essential conversations either fail to begin or are prematurely shut down. Although some treatment options exist, patients may never become aware of them due to these negative patient-provider interactions.

2.3 Provider related factors

Within the broader healthcare system, there are many barriers to advancing sexual medicine education at the training level. Gaps in education begin in medical school, where providers-in-training receive limited exposure to female sexual health. One study found that only about 50% of accredited US medical schools require formal training in sexual medicine, with 20% of medical students receiving no sexual medicine education. Moreover, the same study found that the training provided has been described as inconsistent in method, duration, and content [11]. This contributes to a lack of comfort and confidence when discussing these topics with patients. This raises concerns about the preparedness of graduates to address female sexual health upon entering residency [12].

"I find it genuinely difficult to speak confidently about female sexual dysfunction, largely because it received minimal coverage in our curriculum. In discussing this with peers, it's clear that many of us share the same sentiment. Given its complexity and the profound impact it can have on a patient's quality of life, this lack of emphasis feels like a significant gap in our education."

- Medical student at Drexel University, Class of 2026.

During residency, even specialties directly involved in treating FSD report inadequate preparation. A 2016 review found that only a few residency programs included sexual medicine objectives, defined very generally. Notably, training in OB/GYN involves knowledge in infertility, menopause, high-risk sexual behavior, and skills such as taking a sexual history, while the OB/GYN subspecialty of urogynecology emphasizes pelvic floor dysfunction [13]. One survey found that two-thirds of OB/GYN residents considered sexual health training at large a priority in residency, yet less than 50% were able to describe sexual function disorders or discuss common medications that affect sexual functioning [14]. In the same study, resident performance correlated with greater exposure to didactic sexual health training.

Even postresidency, in specialties such as gynecology, urology, and urogynecology, providers remain dissatisfied with their training in FSD. A survey of urogynecology providers reported that only 71% of these providers felt comfortable treating sexual dysfunction, and 50% found their training in this topic unsatisfactory [13]. Although there are screening tools available, one survey identified that many urogynecology and reconstructive pelvic surgery (URPS) providers underutilize them and often underestimate FSD prevalence; only 22% report consistent screening [13]. The same article identified that some training opportunities exist through professional societies or CME credits, but these require self-motivation and may be inaccessible to many providers.

Even when patients overcome barriers of access and provider training, the process of establishing a clear diagnosis and obtaining appropriate treatment remains fraught. Diagnostic ambiguity, inconsistent clinical guidelines, and regulatory hurdles all converge to constrain the effective management of FSD.

3. Regulatory and policy barriers

The etiology of FSD is multifactorial in nature and spans biological, psychological, and sociocultural domains, often without a singular underlying physiologic cause, which complicates diagnosis and can prolong treatment. Clinicians must assess a broad spectrum of symptoms, including low desire, diminished arousal, anorgasmia, and pain [15]. Accurate diagnosis is further hindered by ambiguity in definitions, the absence of standardized measurement tools, and discrepancies between patient-reported outcomes (PROs) and clinical assessments [16]. Care for FSD remains suboptimal, in part due to limited provider training in diagnostic tools and inconsistencies in treatment approaches [17]. Comorbidities can also obscure diagnosis, and patients with complex presentations may be less likely to disclose symptoms during routine care [18]. Moreover, diagnostic frameworks such as DSM-5 and ICD-11 differ in their classification of FSD [19], creating additional obstacles for regulatory approval and insurance coverage. These classification differences, combined with the multifaceted nature of FSD, contribute to variability in clinical evaluation and highlight the need to examine inconsistencies in diagnostic approaches across specialties and guidelines.

3.1 Diagnostic inconsistencies

The diagnosis and treatment of FSD often involve multiple specialties, including primary care, gynecology, urology, sex therapy, and female pelvic medicine reconstructive surgery [20]. A gynecologist or urologist often emphasizes physical examinations or laboratory testing, whereas a psychologist and other mental health providers focus on psychological assessment and psychotherapy. Laboratory testing should be tailored to specific concerns (e.g., hormonal assays), but such tests are not uniformly diagnostic for FSD. No universally agreed-upon laboratory panel for FSD exists [21]. Because no single physiologic diagnostic test exists for FSD, cross-specialty diagnostic consistency is difficult to achieve [22]. This absence of diagnostic consensus undermines a universally accepted treatment pathway and can delay patient access to appropriate care.

Comorbidities add significant complexity to diagnosing FSD, often creating diagnostic ambiguity. For example, women with diabetes at any age face an elevated risk of FSD [18]. In type 1 diabetes, FSD is frequently associated with depression and anxiety [23], making it difficult to disentangle whether dysfunction arises from diabetes itself, its neurovascular impact on sexual physiology [24], comorbid depression, or medication effects. Mental health conditions further complicate assessment: women have nearly twice the lifetime prevalence of depression and most anxiety disorders compared to men [25], and antidepressants may exert both positive and negative effects on arousal. Relational and sociocultural contributors, including relationship discord, partner sexual dysfunction, life stage stressors, and cultural or religious messaging, add an additional layer of diagnostic variability [3]. These overlapping etiologies underscore the importance of provider awareness of the bidirectional relationship between mental health and FSD, as well as the need for transparent discussions with patients beginning antidepressant therapy.

Beyond comorbidities, inconsistencies in diagnostic frameworks and guidelines introduce further barriers. The DSM-5 reclassified FSD by merging female sexual arousal and desire disorders into a single diagnosis [26], whereas the ICD-10 and ICD-11 continue to separate these diagnoses [19]. Surveys suggest mental health professionals often favor ICD coding for administrative purposes, yet these inconsistencies undermine prognostic clarity and treatment planning [27]. The ICD-11 further consolidated diverse etiologies of sexual dysfunction into one category to facilitate a biopsychosocial approach, but this shift may complicate insurance coverage and encourage pharmacologic or surgical interventions in cases where sexual therapy would be more appropriate [19, 28].

Professional society guidelines are similarly inconsistent: ACOG and ISSWSH recommend compassionate, nonjudgmental inquiry with broad-to-specific questioning [29, 30], while APA guidelines align more rigidly with DSM-5 terminology [31]. Such variation across manuals and societies may lead to differences in patient disclosure, diagnostic labeling, and treatment pathways.

3.2 FDA approval and cost reimbursement

Even when diagnostic criteria are met, patients and providers face systemic barriers in navigating treatment approval and affordability. The FDA approval process, inconsistent insurance coverage, and high out-of-pocket costs collectively limit access to available therapies. Preventive care and education are as important as treatment, yet care for FSD often involves multiple referrals, providers, and therapies. Providers may hesitate to prescribe effective treatments if costs exceed what patients can afford. For example, flibanserin can cost around $830 out of pocket and $20–$25 with insurance coverage, depending on the plan [32]. Comparisons of healthcare utilization show that women with HSDD incur, on average, $1,146 more in annual medical expenses than women without the diagnosis [33]. Additionally, some forms of therapy may not be indicated for certain presentations of FSD, creating further out-of-pocket costs [27].

Medicare and Medicaid coverage of FSD varies. Medicare now covers prescriptions for severe dyspareunia due to menopause under Part D [34]. In comparison, Medicaid coverage differs by state and often focuses on reproductive health (e.g., family planning, sexually transmitted infections) [29]. Additional requirements for off-label use, such as for comorbid diabetes, may further impede access [23].

Regulatory processes also create barriers. The FDA historically emphasizes PROs over clinician assessments and has assigned FSD review to the Division of Urology, which may be suboptimal because FSD involves multiple systems beyond the urogenital tract [30]. Boxed warnings, such as those for low-dose vaginal estrogen, can create provider and patient hesitation despite limited endometrial risk [17, 35]. FDA approval is based on safety and efficacy for specific indications rather than the mechanism of action. Flibanserin, initially developed for major depressive disorder, failed in that indication but demonstrated increased libido as an off-target effect [36]. Even with approval, prior authorization requirements and Risk Evaluation and Mitigation Strategies (REMS) necessitate provider certification and pharmacist involvement, creating time and logistical barriers [17, 32]. Out-of-pocket costs can vary widely, from approximately $100 per month without insurance to $25 with coverage.

These regulatory, insurance, and cost barriers highlight the fragility of the clinical pathway for FSD and underscore how access to approved treatments can be constrained by systemic and procedural hurdles. They also reflect deeper limitations in the scientific foundation itself, including preclinical models, study designs, and outcome measures that ultimately determine which interventions reach patients.

4. Scientific and translational barriers

Even with improved access and clearer regulatory guidance, evidence-based interventions for FSD remain limited. Research in sexual medicine faces methodological, conceptual, and practical hurdles that constrain the development of effective treatments. Challenges include study design complexities, recruitment limitations, outcome measure selection, and the historically male-centric perspective in sexual function research. This section explores how these scientific and experimental barriers affect both our understanding of FSD and the translation of research findings into clinical care, highlighting the ongoing need for rigorous and nuanced investigation.

4.1 Translational pipeline challenges

The translational pathway from preclinical studies to clinical trials presents unique challenges in FSD. Existing animal models fail to capture the relational and sociocultural dimensions of human sexuality, and physiologic assessments are often limited by the need for anesthesia. As a result, early-stage findings are difficult to translate into meaningful therapies for patients. For a treatment to be approved by the FDA, it must go through a series of rigorous studies to establish its safety and efficacy. The process begins with preclinical research. Generally, this refers to animal studies to assess feasibility (e.g., dosing, toxicity, tolerability). There have been a range of animal models for female sexual function over the years, including rodents, primates, and even birds [37]. The choice of animal depends on what methodological approach is being used to evaluate sexual function (e.g., behavioral vs. neurophysiologic endpoints). Behavioral models of sexual function are well established in rodents, but they cannot fully capture the relational, cognitive, and cultural components that influence human sexual function. Physiologic models, which aim to measure manifestations such as pain, genital arousal, or anorgasmia, often require anesthesia during testing, which disrupts neural signaling and confounds results, limiting their translational relevance. All animal studies require careful interpretation when extrapolating results to humans. Thus, while preclinical studies are a necessary step for understanding mechanisms and safety, they are inherently insufficient to capture the full complexity of human sexual function, underscoring the need for carefully designed clinical trials.

The subsequent steps in the regulatory process involve clinical studies in increasingly larger cohorts. Broadly speaking, these studies begin with a small (10–20 participants) Phase I study, often termed a "first in human" study. These initial clinical trials are designed as a first screening test to assess safety, typically in healthy controls. Phases II and III are conducted in the target patient population and evaluate efficacy in addition to safety in cohorts ranging from hundreds to thousands of participants. The average success rate across all drug classes, from an initial investigational new drug (IND) application to a likelihood of approval (LOA) from the FDA, is 10.4% [38]. Unfortunately, there are not enough data to calculate metrics on successful transitions from Phase I to LOA for medications specifically for sexual dysfunction. The low success rate is reflected by the limited number of drugs approved for women over the past decade: just two (Addyi and Vyleesi). Careful and rigorous clinical study design is therefore essential to meet FDA-defined endpoints for approval, helping to avoid the substantial costs of Phase II or III trials that might otherwise lead to product abandonment. For female sexual function studies, additional methodological barriers regarding study execution complicate the design and conduct of a rigorous clinical trial.

There are many methodological challenges to conducting clinical studies in FSD that raise the question of ecological validity. Physiological measurements, such as vaginal photoplethysmography (VPP), usually take place in environments such as laboratories or clinics that are not conducive to replicating a natural setting that reflects real-world sexual experience. Descending cortical pathways inhibit sexual arousal and are strengthened by the artificial or clinical setting in which sexual arousal would be inappropriate [39]. To overcome this inhibition, researchers use sexual stimuli, such as erotic visual or auditory stimuli. It becomes a catch-22: stimuli should reflect participants' preferences, but standardization is required for cross-participant comparisons. Past research has indicated that stimuli choice may not have a significant effect on genital arousal [40], but the same cannot be said for subjective arousal. Ensuring concordance between objective genital measures and subjective reports is critical, as misalignment could obscure true treatment effects and reduce the likelihood that the FDA considers a therapy clinically meaningful [41].

Another important factor to consider in clinical trial design for FSD is recruitment. Many women are uncomfortable with the invasiveness of the testing equipment (e.g., VPP) or with being exposed to erotic visual or auditory stimuli [42]. This self-selection bias leads to samples that may not be representative of the broader population with FSD. Additionally, factors such as lack of education on sexual health (e.g., not recognizing dysfunction as a medical issue), body shaming or other negative messaging, interpersonal relationship dynamics, privacy concerns, and religious or cultural beliefs could prevent someone from participating. This can skew data toward participants who are more comfortable with these aspects [42]. These challenges are not just methodological but also cultural and social, creating unique recruitment barriers.

4.2 Outcome measurement limitations

Selecting appropriate outcome measures remains one of the most persistent challenges in FSD research. Heavy reliance on PROs introduces variability, while physiological tools such as VPP face methodological and interpretive limitations. This misalignment complicates both trial design and regulatory approval.
A central challenge in designing a clinical study for FSD is choosing the primary outcome measure. FSD is multifaceted and often presents with multiple symptoms, making it difficult to select a single quantitative metric to evaluate efficacy. For example, if targeting female sexual interest/arousal disorder, the study team would have to decide between metrics such as genital vasocongestion, sexual desire, frequency of satisfying sexual events, or even quality of life. Typically, this decision is made in consultation with the FDA when seeking regulatory guidance for a new drug or device.

Each possible outcome measure has distinct advantages and disadvantages. Self-reporting measures have inherent flaws but remain a versatile tool to collect data quickly, especially as many studies include sexual function as a secondary or exploratory objective. They allow researchers who are not experts in sexual function to collect validated data and contribute to overall knowledge. Even after deciding that a PRO would be the most appropriate, researchers must still decide which metric to use. There are many validated surveys for assessing FSD; the most widely used is the Female Sexual Function Index (FSFI) [43]. The FSFI is a 19-item questionnaire that asks respondents to rate their sexual function over the past four weeks in six domains: desire, arousal, lubrication, orgasm, satisfaction, and pain.

If an objective measurement is more appropriate, there are options, but far fewer than surveys and other PROs. VPP, which measures vaginal pulse amplitude, has been the gold standard for measuring genital vasocongestion since the 1990s [44]. It has received criticism for its low concordance with subjective arousal; essentially, it is not reflective of the cognitive experience, which is paramount when it comes to real-world satisfaction [45]. Some researchers are beginning to investigate vulvar blood perfusion using noninvasive methods such as laser Doppler imaging (LDI). Preliminary research suggests improved sexual concordance, which would make vulvar blood perfusion a more appropriate metric for clinical trial endpoints [46]. There are other, less common ways to measure sexual function, including pH or chemical indicator strips to assess lubrication, heart rate variability, and skin conductance [47]. However, they are not as popular because of limited validation, poor specificity, or participant burden.

4.3 Research infrastructure issues

The study of FSD has long been shaped by structural disadvantages. Sexual medicine has historically prioritized male function, leaving women's sexual health with fewer resources, limited expertise, and underdeveloped training pathways. These gaps have persisted, slowing progress and shaping which questions are asked and which therapies are pursued. Much of what we have discussed so far – laboratory design, measurement challenges, and study conditions – operates at the micro level. However, broader forces, rooted in the historical and ongoing male-centered orientation of medicine and academia, continue to influence the field.

Research is also inherently expensive, and the allocation of funding has reinforced these disparities. Even the largest funding mechanisms have traditionally favored studies of male sexual function, while women's sexual health has received proportionally less support. This has affected everything from the types of interventions tested to the availability of clinical expertise, highlighting how deeply structural and historical factors shape the trajectory of research in FSD.

5. Discussion

Patients experiencing FSD face many barriers in accessing care from the perspectives of clinical intervention, policy, and research. It is important, as a society, to improve awareness about sexual health to reduce stigma and empower people to seek care when necessary. In clinical environments broadly, the inconsistent and often insufficient quality of care requires vast improvement. While limited in scope, existing clinical recommendations for treating FSD patients must be more widely adopted. Providers and trainees across specialties need more exposure to and training in FSD care to support their patients' treatment and well-being. It is essential to rebuild trust with patients who have been repeatedly dismissed by providers whose knowledge to treat their concerns is limited.

In developing evidence-based clinical practice, accessibility for patients must be considered. Treatments cannot be effective if they never reach the patients they aim to help. Initial FDA approval needs to place greater value on the experiences and recommendations of clinicians in moving toward approval. Once approved, insurance companies must lower the barrier to access to care by trusting knowledgeable providers to determine what is medically necessary. Prior to reaching the phase of FDA approval, preclinical and clinical research face distinct challenges that need attention. FSD is uniquely challenging to study and requires physiological, biopsychosocial consideration. Developing novel, creative methods that maximize the accuracy of their data requires appropriate resources, approvals, and logistical improvements. Research funding for FSD should be prioritized, as male sexual function is, which would provide FSD researchers with the resources to develop novel and effective treatment options with compelling evidence to validate them.

6. Conclusion

Taken together, these barriers form a tightly linked chain: limited clinical infrastructure restricts access, diagnostic and regulatory inconsistencies obstruct care even when patients reach specialists, and scientific limitations slow the development of new therapies. Progress will require a coordinated approach that spans training, diagnostic consensus, regulatory reform, and sustained research investment. Only by addressing these interconnected challenges can the field of sexual medicine begin to close the persistent gap in care for women with FSD.

DOI: http://dx.doi.org/10.5772/intechopen.1013125

Acknowledgments

We would like to thank Drs. Cramer and Darrow for their roles as Principal Investigators of the Restorative Neurotrauma Lab, and Dr. Netoff for his role as Principal Investigator of the Neural Netoff Laboratory. Thank you to Drs. Satish Vitta and Padma Satish for their valuable advice and support. We are grateful to Arjun Ramachandran for taking the time to talk about his experience with medical education and provide feedback about the curriculum.

Author details

Elizabeth C. Bottorff[1,2]*, Ava G. Grotting[2] and Srinidhi Satish[2]

1 Biomedical Engineering Department, University of Minnesota, Minneapolis, United States

2 Department of Neurosurgery, Hennepin Healthcare Research Institute, Minneapolis, United States

*Address all correspondence to: bottorff@umn.edu

References

[1] Stanley EE, Pope RJ. Characteristics of female sexual health programs and providers in the United States. Sexual Medicine. 2022;**10**(4):100524–100524

[2] Stanley EE, Pfoh E, Lipold L, Martinez K.Gap in sexual dysfunction management between male and female patients seen in primary care: An observational study. Journal of General Internal Medicine. 2025;**40**(4):847–853

[3] Brotto LA, Bitzer J, Laan E, Leiblum S, Luria M.Women's sexual desire and arousal disorders. The Journal of Sexual Medicine. 2010;7(1):586–614

[4] Harsh V, McGarvey EL, Clayton AH.Physician attitudes regarding hypoactive sexual desire disorder in a primary care clinic: A pilot study. The Journal of Sexual Medicine. 2008;**5**(3):640–645

[5] Scavello I, Maseroli E, Di Stasi V, Vignozzi L.Sexual Health in Menopause. Medicina. 2019;**55**(9):559

[6] Nelson KM, Gray A, Haiken S, Underhill K.The state of sexual education: State laws and regulations mandating sexual education in the United States. American Journal of Public Health. 2025;**115**(10):1723–1733

[7] Lindau ST, Tetteh AS, Kasza K, Gilliam M.What schools teach our patients about sex: Content, quality, and influences on sex education. Obstetrics & Gynecology. 2008;**111**(2):256–266

[8] Hall KS, Moreau C, Trussell J.Lower use of sexual and reproductive health services among women with frequent religious participation, regardless of sexual experience. Journal of Women's Health. 2012;**21**(7):739–747

[9] Berman L, Berman J, Felder S, Pollets D, Chhabra S, Miles M, et al. Seeking help for sexual function complaints: What gynecologists need to know about the female patient's experience. Fertility and Sterility 2003;**79**:572–576

[10] Goldstein I, Lines C, Pyke R, Scheld JS.National differences in patient–clinician communication regarding hypoactive sexual desire disorder. The Journal of Sexual Medicine. 2009;**6**(5):1349–1357

[11] Beebe S, Payne N, Posid T, Diab D, Horning P, Scimeca A, et al. The lack of sexual health education in medical training leaves students and residents feeling unprepared. The Journal of Sexual Medicine 2021;**18**:1998–2004

[12] Prize NBT, Kanat SS, Wruble ACKW.Gaps in sexual health content of healthcare professional curriculum: A systematic review of educational interventions. BMC Medical Education. 2023;**23**(1):926

[13] Ward SA, Cornely RM, Mendiola M, Royce CS, Winkelman WD, Hacker MR, et al. Education in female sexual function and dysfunction among American urogynecologic society members: An unmet need. Southern Medical Journal 2024;**117**:7–10

[14] Worly B, Manriquez M, Stagg A, Blanchard MH, Ogburn T, Carson SA, et al. Sexual health education in obstetrics and gynecology (Ob-Gyn) Residencies—A resident physician

survey. The Journal of Sexual Medicine 2021;**18**:1042–1052

[15] Parish SJ, Pope R.Female sexual health. Obstetrics and Gynecology Clinics of North America. 2024;**51**(2):223–239

[16] Imprialos KP, Koutsampasopoulos K, Katsimardou A, Bouloukou S, Theodoulidis I, Themistoklis M, et al. Female Sexual dysfunction: A problem hidden in the shadows. Current Pharmaceutical Design 2021;**27**:3762–3774

[17] Kingsberg SA, Schaffir J, Faught BM, Pinkerton JV, Parish SJ, Iglesia CB, et al. Female sexual health: Barriers to optimal outcomes and a roadmap for improved patient–clinician communications. Journal of Women's Health 2019;**28**:432–443

[18] Bitzer J, Giraldi A, Pfaus J.Sexual desire and hypoactive sexual desire disorder in women. Introduction and overview. Standard Operating Procedure (SOP Part 1). The Journal of Sexual Medicine. 2013;**10**(1):36–49

[19] Başar K The changes in ICD-11 related to sexual health and dysfunction and their implication for clinical practice. Turkish Journal of Psychiatry [Internet]. 2024 Available from: https://turkpsikiyatri.com/submission/MakaleKontrol?Id=VFdwak1VNVVhejA9 [Accessed: 2025-September-18]

[20] Shoureshi PS, Dubinskaya A, Bresee C, Karram M, Eilber KS. Female sexual dysfunction: Lack of change in physician practice patterns over time. Gynecology and Pelvic Medicine. 2024;**7**:1–1

[21] Sexual Dysfunction Disorders in Women | Women's Health [Internet]. Available from: https://www.youtube.com/watch?v=GXTQNkdZOMo [Accessed: 2025-September-16]

[22] Elanjian AI, Kammo S, Braman L, Liaw A.Advancing women's health: a scoping review of pharmaceutical therapies for female sexual dysfunction. Sexes. 2025;**6**(3):38

[23] Enzlin P, Rosen R, Wiegel M, Brown J, Wessells H, Gatcomb P, et al. Sexual dysfunction in women with type 1 diabetes: Long-term findings from the DCCT/ EDIC study cohort. Diabetes Care 2009;**32**:780–785

[24] Basson R, Gilks T. Women's sexual dysfunction associated with psychiatric disorders and their treatment. Womens Health. 2018;**14**:1–16

[25] Altemus M, Sarvaiya N, Neill Epperson C.Sex differences in anxiety and depression clinical perspectives. Frontiers in Neuroendocrinology. 2014;**35**(3):320–330

[26] Sungur MZ, Gündüz A. A comparison of DSM-IV-TR and DSM-5 definitions for sexual dysfunctions: critiques and challenges. The Journal of Sexual Medicine. 2014;**11**(2):364–373

[27] First MB, Rebello TJ, Keeley JW, Bhargava R, Dai Y, Kulygina M, et al. Do mental health professionals use diagnostic classifications the way we think they do? A global survey. World Psychiatry 2018;**17**:187–195

[28] Smith D. Women and sex: What is "dysfunctional"? Monitor on Psychology. Internet. 2003;**34**(4). https://www-apa-org.ezp2.lib.umn.edu/monitor/apr03/women

[29] Parish SJ, Hahn SR, Goldstein SW, Giraldi A, Kingsberg SA, Larkin L, et al. The international society for the study of women's sexual health process of care for the identification of sexual concerns and problems in Women. Mayo Clinic Proceedings 2019;**94**:842–856

[30] Armstrong C.ACOG guideline on sexual dysfunction in women. American Family Physician. 2011;**84**(6):705–709

[31] American Psychiatric Association. Diagnostic and Statistical Manual of Mental Disorders. Fifth Edition. [Internet]. American Psychiatric Association; 2013 Available from: https://psychiatryonline.org/DOI/book/10.1176/appi.books.9780890425596 [Accessed: 2025-September-18]

[32] Holt H, Tingen J.Flibanserin (Addyi) for hypoactive sexual desire disorder in Premenopausal Women. American Family Physician. 2016;**93**(10):826

[33] Foley K, Foley D, Johnson BH. Healthcare resource utilization and expenditures of women diagnosed with hypoactive sexual desire disorder. Journal of Medical Economics. 2010;**13**(4):583–590

[34] Dyspareunia: CMS Clarification Results In Expanded Treatment And Coverage Under Medicare Part D. PR Newswire [Internet]. 2018 May 10; Available from: https://www.prnewswire.com/news-releases/dyspareunia-cms-clarification-results-in-expanded-treatment-and-coverage-under-medicare-part-d-300646627.html?tc=eml_cleartime [Accessed: 2025-September-18]

[35] Manson JE, Goldstein SR, Kagan R, Kaunitz AM, Liu JH, Pinkerton JV, et al. Why the product labeling for low-dose vaginal estrogen should be changed. Menopause 2014;**21**:911–916

[36] Pierrelus C, Patel P, Carlson K Flibanserin. In: StatPearls [Internet]. Treasure Island (FL): StatPearls Publishing; 2025. Available from: http://www.ncbi.nlm.nih.gov/books/NBK589649/ [Accessed: 2025-September-18]

[37] Marson L, Giamberardino MA, Costantini R, Czakanski P, Wesselmann U.Animal models for the study of female sexual dysfunction. Sexual Medicine Reviews. 2013;**1**(2):108–122

[38] Hay M, Thomas DW, Craighead JL, Economides C, Rosenthal J.Clinical development success rates for investigational drugs. Nature Biotechnology. 2014;**32**(1):40–51

[39] Katz MA, Penniston TL, Barry C, Micanovic N, Seto MC, Chivers ML. Use of sexual stimuli in research and clinical settings: Expert opinion and recommendations. Sexual Medicine. 2023;**11**(2):1–10

[40] Chivers ML, Seto MC, Blanchard R.Gender and sexual orientation differences in sexual response to sexual activities versus gender of actors in sexual films. Journal of Personality and Social Psychology. 2007;**93**(6):1108–1121

[41] Meston CM, Stanton AM. Understanding sexual arousal and subjective–genital arousal desynchrony in women. Nature Reviews Urology. 2019;**16**(2):107–120

[42] Huberman JS, McInnis MK, Bouchard KN, Dawson SJ, Pukall CF, Chivers ML.Exploring comfort levels and the role of compensation in sexual

psychophysiology study participation. Archives of Sexual Behavior. 2019;**48**(8):2389–2402

[43] Rosen C, Brown J, Heiman S, Leib R.The Female Sexual Function Index (FSFI): A multidimensional self-report instrument for the assessment of female sexual function. Journal of Sex & Marital Therapy. 2000;**26**(2):191–208

[44] Laan E, Everaerd W. Physiological measures of vaginal vasocongestion. International Journal of Impotence Research. 1998;**10**(Suppl 2):S107–110. discussion S124-125

[45] Chivers ML, Seto MC, Lalumière ML, Laan E, Grimbos T. Agreement of self-reported and genital measures of sexual arousal in Men and Women: A meta-analysis. Archives of Sexual Behavior. 2010;**39**(1):5–56

[46] Bouchard KN, Pukall CF Validation of laser Doppler flowmetry for the continuous measurement of women's genital response. Psychophysiology [Internet]. 2022 Dec 7; Available from: https://onlinelibrary.wiley.com/DOI/10.1111/psyp.14230 [Accessed: 2023-April-1]

[47] Kukkonen TM.Devices and methods to measure female sexual arousal. Sexual Medicine Reviews. 2015;**3**(4):225–244

Chapter 2

Misinformation on Digital Platforms about the Use of Medicinal Plants and Herbal Medicines: The Search for Managing Climacteric Symptoms

Ana Claudia F. Amaral, Débora de Castro Soares, Diogo A. Folly, Jefferson R. A. Silva and Elaine Cristina Ferreira Dias

Abstract

This study investigates the dissemination of information on the use of medicinal plants and herbal medicines for managing climacteric symptoms, with a particular emphasis on the risks posed by health misinformation circulating through digital social networks. The chapter aims to critically analyze content shared on these platforms, contrasting it with official, evidence-based guidelines in women's health. Methodologically, the project employed a mixed-methods design, combining quantitative and qualitative approaches with digital ethnography to map content related to recommended treatments for climacteric symptoms and to perform a documentary analysis against the official recommendations of the Brazilian Ministry of Health. The findings revealed a broad circulation of unverified information, frequently disseminated by institutional profiles and digital influencers, endorsing medicinal plants and herbal medicines for climacteric management. Expanding access to trustworthy information, whether through media outlets, digital platforms, or community settings, is crucial to strengthening society's capacity to distinguish between reliable data and misleading claims. Fostering a culture that values scientific knowledge, while promoting closer collaboration among health institutions, educators, and civil society, represents an essential step toward building a more critical, informed, and resilient society in the face of health misinformation

Keywords: natural products, health communication, menopause management, social media influence, digital media

1. Introduction

The climacteric period corresponds to a natural phase characterized by a progressive reduction in ovarian activity and the consequent decline in estrogen production, generally occurring between the ages of 35 and 60, marking the transition from a woman's fertile phase to her non-reproductive period [1]. This transition encompasses the phases of perimenopause, menopause, and postmenopause and is marked by significant hormonal changes, including decreased levels of estrogen and progesterone, which play essential roles in reproductive health, bone metabolism, cardiovascular function, and emotional balance [2, 3].

Estrogen plays a central role in regulating the menstrual cycle, promoting endometrial thickening and ovarian follicle maturation. During the reproductive phase, this process occurs through the coordinated interaction between hormones produced by the hypothalamus, pituitary gland, and ovaries. In the follicular phase, estrogen levels reach their peak, preparing the body for ovulation. Menopause, defined as the cessation of menstruation for at least 12 consecutive months, involves a sharp decline in this hormone, leading to various symptoms that may negatively impact women's well-being [1–3].

The hormonal decline characteristic of the climacteric period is associated with symptoms such as hot flashes, sleep disturbances, vaginal dryness, mood changes, bone mass loss, joint pain, weight gain, and cognitive impairment. In addition to these physical effects, emotional and social issues are also intensified, as women's aging is still frequently perceived as a loss of social value, attractiveness, and productivity [4, 5].

According to data from the 2022 Census, Brazil has, for the first time in its history, registered a greater number of women compared to men. Among the country's total population of 203,062,512 inhabitants, over 51% are women. Approximately 26% of these women are within the 40 to 55 age group, highlighting the significant proportion of women who are likely experiencing the climacteric period in Brazil [6].

In certain situations, a treatment aimed specifically at managing climacteric symptoms may be recommended. Options range from pharmacological treatments, both hormonal and non-hormonal, to complementary therapies. Although hormone therapy has been shown to alleviate symptoms such as hot flashes and insomnia, it is linked to potential adverse effects, including an elevated risk of thromboembolic events and hormone-dependent cancers, such as breast and endometrial cancers [7]. Due to these limitations, alternative therapeutic approaches, particularly the use of natural compounds and medicinal plants, have gained attention. These alternatives are valued for their effectiveness and safety profile, as evidenced by recent research on phytotherapies during the climacteric period [8].

During the climacteric period, there is a growing interest in medicinal plants and herbal therapies. These are often promoted as natural, risk-free alternatives. However, scientific evidence does not always support this perception of unrestricted safety. The belief that natural products are harmless can lead to indiscriminate use, particularly in countries such as Brazil, where self-medication is common. According to data from the National Survey on Access and Use of Medicines, over 16% of the Brazilian population uses medications without professional guidance and frequently uses plant-based products without proper prescriptions. This reality underscores the importance of making informed decisions and receiving professional monitoring, even when using alternative therapies [9].

This concern is further amplified in the digital environment. In cyberspace, there is a growing circulation of content about health and treatments that has not undergone scientific validation. Social media platforms have been used by influencers, unregulated therapists, and people without technical training to promote supposed natural solutions or treatments, which contribute to the spread of inaccurate and misleading information. In many cases, these discourses exploit the appeal of "folk wisdom" and "natural remedies," attracting especially those seeking alternatives to effective treatments, even if they are not based on reliable evidence [10].

The challenge of misinformation extends beyond national borders. A broader perspective is offered by the Truth Quest study, conducted by the Organization for Economic Co-operation and Development (OECD) in 2024, involving 21 countries, which investigated how individuals perceive true and false news. Findings suggest that, on average, people correctly identify the veracity of about 60% of the news they consume. However, given that a substantial portion of the available information may be false, estimated at around two-thirds, studies suggest that individuals believe approximately 40% of this misleading content. This indicates that a considerable share of the information perceived as accurate is, in fact, incorrect. Country scores varied, with Finland achieving 66% accuracy and Brazil only 54%, highlighting a 12-percentage-point gap. From a regional perspective, Nordic countries such as Finland and Norway performed best, while Latin American nations, particularly Brazil and Colombia, demonstrated the greatest need for improvement [11].

The impact of health misinformation is especially pronounced in Brazil. Data from the Ministry of Science, Technology, and Innovations indicate that 78% of Brazilians use social media as their primary source of health information. Furthermore, the 2023 Public Perception of Science and Technology Survey reveals a concerning scenario regarding the spread of misinformation: five out of ten Brazilians report frequently encountering news that appears to be false (50.8%). These figures highlight the severity of the fake news problem and its potential influence on society [12].

Primary health care (PHC) has, in principle, the role of comprehensively addressing the needs of women at all stages of life, including menopause. However, there is a significant gap in care for this population, marked by the absence of widely adopted clinical protocols and insufficient training of professionals to deal with the symptoms and demands of this phase. Although menopause is covered in guidelines and public policies outside the field of women's health, in practice, care continues to focus on maternal and child health, which contributes to the invisibility of women transitioning to menopause within basic health services [3].

Furthermore, prevailing approaches to menstruation tend to restrict the experiences of cisgender women, marginalizing transmasculine and non-binary people who also have ovaries and experience hormonal and physiological changes during this period. This invisibility compromises the effectiveness of care and reinforces the exclusion of identities that do not fit into cis-heteronormative norms, both in health services and in academic production on the subject. The invisibility of this population contributes to even greater neglect in health services and in the production of scientific knowledge about their demands [10].

In this context, this study seeks to critically assess the information disseminated on social media regarding the use of herbal medicines and medicinal plants for the management of climacteric symptoms, contrasting it with available scientific evidence and official documents, including the Ministry of Health Guideline for Women's Care during the Climacteric [3].

In addition, this study seeks to discuss the impacts of health misinformation and self-medication, as well as highlight the importance of scientific communication and inclusive public policies.

1.1 Climacteric treatments and management symptoms

The climacteric is a natural phenomenon that signals the gradual end of the reproductive phase in the lives of people with ovaries, usually occurring between the ages of 45 and 55, although this range may vary. It is not only a biological process but also a social and symbolic one, influenced by cultural and historical aspects. This transition is marked by a progressive reduction in ovarian hormones, especially estrogen and progesterone, whose decline is associated with changes involving the menstrual cycle but also has repercussions on cardiovascular, bone, metabolic, and emotional health [13].

The climacteric period is traditionally divided into three phases: perimenopause, menopause, and postmenopause. Perimenopause is marked by hormonal changes and irregular menstrual cycles. Menopause is clinically identified after twelve consecutive months without menstruation. Postmenopause is a period in which ovarian hormones remain at persistently low levels. The postmenopausal phase is associated with an increased risk of various conditions, including osteoporosis, sarcopenia, mood swings, cognitive impairment, and an increased risk of cardiovascular disease [2, 14].

Estrogen is a hormone that is essential for physiological balance throughout the reproductive phase. Its action extends to the thickening of the endometrium, vaginal lubrication, preservation of bone mineral density, regulation of cardiovascular function, and modulation of neurotransmitters related to emotional well-being. With the progressive reduction of estrogen levels during menopause, it is common to experience clinical manifestations such as hot flashes, night sweats, insomnia, fatigue, anxiety, depression, decreased libido, pain during sexual intercourse, and difficulties with memory and attention [1, 4].

More than just a biological process, menopause is part of a sociocultural fabric marked by stigmas that link women's aging to a loss of attractiveness, productivity, and social value. These beliefs reinforce the silence surrounding menopause and intensify the subjective suffering experienced during this period. In addition, these demands are rendered invisible in health services, which often disregard the emotional and social complexities associated with the climacteric transition [10].

The most appropriate treatment for climacteric symptoms should consider the clinical profile, risk factors, and specific characteristics of each patient. Therapeutic approaches may include hormonal, non-hormonal, or a combination of both options, always accompanied by guidance on lifestyle changes. Regular physical activity, a balanced diet, and giving up bad habits are essential components for improving quality of life and reducing climacteric symptoms [2,14].

The Guideline for Women Care during the Climacteric emphasizes the importance of recognizing women as protagonists of their own journey, ensuring access to information and professional support that enable informed decisions on how to experience this stage of life. It also acknowledges herbal medicine as one of the therapeutic options, providing specific standardization and dosage recommendations for only six herbal medicines, along with their potential side effects and contraindications [3].

Herbal medicines are defined as those obtained exclusively from active plant-based raw materials, whose safety and efficacy are supported by clinical evidence, and which are characterized by consistent quality. According to Brazilian health regulations, these products cannot contain active ingredients that are isolated or synthesized in a laboratory, even if they are of plant origin. Anvisa's Resolution RDC No. 26/2014 establishes criteria to classify and control these medicines, distinguishing them from other formulations containing isolated natural compounds [3].

Phytotherapy became more relevant as an integrative practice in the Unified Health System (*Sistema Único de Saúde* – SUS) in the 2000s, especially after the creation of the National Policy on Medicinal Plants and Herbal Medicines in 2006. This initiative was followed, in 2008, by the implementation of a national program that supported its execution. These legal instruments establish guidelines to expand population access to treatments based on specific natural resources, fostering the integration of traditional knowledge with scientific therapeutic approaches in the context of public health. Since then, local initiatives providing phytotherapy within health services have continued to expand [3].

Despite advances in public policies focused on women's health, the clinical management of menopause still relies on outdated guidelines, such as the Ministry of Health Guideline published in 2008. This limitation reflects a model of care strongly centered on biomedical aspects, with little consideration for the emotional, social, and subjective dimensions that shape this stage of life. Several studies indicate that, in most services, care for menopausal women remains fragmented and insufficiently responsive to their broader needs [10].

1.2 Misinformation and health risks on digital platforms

The Economic and Social Forum has identified misinformation, driven by the intensive use of information and communication technologies, as one of the ten major trends in networked society. Technological advances enable the spread of fake news across digital platforms, especially social media, on an almost uncontrollable scale and speed, with unpredictable consequences [15].

This informational chaos can be classified into three types of informational disorder:

Disinformation: misinformation created with the intention of confusing, provoking doubt, or embedding hate speech.

Misinformation: misinformation shared unintentionally can cause misunderstandings, such as statistical errors or captions that do not match the content, creating false connections.

Malinformation: news with a factual basis that is modified and taken out of context with the intention of misinforming, such as leaking private information into the public sphere.

The pandemic has exacerbated this disorder, affecting public understanding of vaccines, and digital media, such as social networks, have become the main source of misinformation. The importance of health information, as well as the obstacles arising from limited health literacy, has become evident. There are also difficulties related to the consumption of digital information, which often neglects the needs of patients. This can result in the selective evaluation of health content shared online, which reinforces misconceptions and gaps in understanding [15, 16].

During the COVID-19 pandemic, coordination between public health institutions and media outlets played a strategic role in combating misinformation. Initiatives such as the production of informative content on official channels, especially on digital platforms such as YouTube, were developed to disseminate accurate guidance and strengthen adherence to vaccination. At the same time, actions aimed at improving the population's digital literacy proved to be fundamental in reducing vulnerability to the consumption and spread of misinformation [5, 17].

According to data from the Ministry of Science, Technology and Innovations (MCTI, 2023), 78% of Brazilians seek health information through digital platforms. Women between the ages of 40 and 65 are among the most frequent users. While these platforms provide easier access to information, they have also become a breeding ground for misinformation, particularly regarding natural therapies and herbal products [18].

The practice of self-medication, which is widespread in Brazil, is reinforced both by difficulties in accessing health services and by cultural factors that associate natural remedies with the idea of absolute safety. This perception, although common, disregards the potential risks associated with the unsupervised use of medicinal plants and herbal remedies, such as allergic reactions, liver toxicity, and dangerous drug interactions. Studies indicate that the population often resorts to these resources without professional guidance, reinforcing the need for more effective educational and regulatory actions [9].

Furthermore, the problem of misinformation about menopause is exacerbated by the erasure experienced by transmasculine and non-binary people. Although they may undergo hormonal changes related to menopause if they have ovaries, their experiences are often disregarded in clinical protocols, institutional discourse, and public policy. This invisibility creates barriers to accessing reliable information and adequate healthcare, perpetuating existing inequalities and further marginalizing these bodies.

In this context, academic studies must contribute critical knowledge that confronts misinformation and promotes evidence-based health education. This knowledge must integrate scientific research, cultural practices, and contemporary demands. Therefore, this theoretical framework is anchored in understanding the intersections of menopause, public health, digital misinformation, self-medication, herbal medicine, and the inclusion of diverse bodies in care practices.

2. Research parameters

The methodological approach adopted was netnography, used to map content related to the recommended treatments for climacteric symptoms. In this context, netnography aims to study human behavior in online environments, considering broader communication factors and mechanisms, such as the dynamics of digital platforms [19].

Thus, the overall objective was to evaluate the indications of treatments for climacteric symptoms shared on digital platforms. The research was structured in three stages: first, identifying the platforms most used by women based on predefined descriptors; second, conducting a literature review on the topic and consulting official health databases, including the Ministry of Health (MH) of Brazil; and third, cross-referencing unofficial content with official MH recommendations on treatments for climacteric symptoms.

In the first stage, YouTube, Instagram, and X (formerly Twitter) channels were mapped using criteria of relevance of views on the theme, identifying (1) the profile of content producers; (2) recommendations and areas of expertise; and (3) number of views. The selection of content was guided by criteria of relevance and reach, considering publications that had at least 10,000 interactions, including views, likes, comments, and shares. The objective of this stage was to map which medicinal plants and herbal medicines are most frequently promoted as alternatives for managing menopausal symptoms, as well as to identify which symptoms are associated with these indications on social media and whether content producers mention the MH guidelines or not.

Based on this analysis, the botanical species most frequently mentioned on social media but not included in the MH guideline were selected for further investigation. This stage also includes a detailed literature review in scientific databases such as PubMed, Scopus, and Google Scholar to verify the existence of studies that support, or do not support, the therapeutic claims associated with these plants.

3. Data collection and analysis procedures

Data collection and analysis were designed to provide a comprehensive and critical understanding of the dissemination of information on the use of medicinal plants and herbal medicines for managing menopausal symptoms, particularly within digital social networks. This approach is justified by the growing relevance of these platforms as sources of health information and by the increasing demand for alternative therapies, often driven by perceived gaps in formal health care services, including primary care.

The data collection process involved systematic monitoring of three widely used platforms: YouTube, Instagram, and X (formerly Twitter), from November 2024 to March 2025. These platforms were selected based on their high number of active users and the significant volume of content related to herbal medicine and menopause.

Selection criteria prioritized posts with broad reach, defined as those with at least 10,000 views. Searches were carried out using specific keywords related to women's health and menopause, such as "medicinal plants for menopause," "herbal medicine for menopause," "natural treatment for menopause," "menopause symptoms," and "natural remedies for menopause."

The collected information was organized into digital spreadsheets and classified by variables, including medicinal plants cited, associated symptoms (e.g., hot flashes, insomnia, depression, vaginal dryness), type of content creator (health professionals, digital influencers, natural therapists, or sales profiles), and references to scientific sources, research articles, technical guidelines, or official institutions such as the Ministry of Health or ANVISA.

Subsequently, a document analysis was performed, comparing social media content with the recommendations outlined in the Guideline for Women's Care during the Climacteric [3].

A comprehensive literature review was also conducted, incorporating national and international studies to assess the level of scientific evidence supporting or refuting the therapeutic claims attributed to these plants. The review encompassed scientific articles, systematic reviews, meta-analyses, and official documents available in databases such as PubMed, Scopus, Google Scholar, and SciELO.

Finally, data analysis employed a triangulation strategy, integrating multiple sources: (1) narratives from social media and (2) official documents, including the Ministry of Health Guideline and related scientific articles. This strategy ensured a critical and evidence-based perspective, enabling both an understanding of misinformation processes in the climacteric context and the identification of treatments supported by scientific evidence.

4. Results

The findings from the survey conducted on digital social networks reveal a widespread dissemination of information about the use of medicinal plants for managing climacteric symptoms. A significant portion of this information lacks formal scientific support or is not aligned with official public health recommendations, such as those in the guideline [3].

Using digital ethnography to systematize the dynamics of content production on the most prominent channels, we identified characteristics of information disseminators on digital platforms. Among the content creators: (1) the majority are women; (2) many are nutritionists and gynecologists; and (3) the predominant channels are related to health, personal care/beauty, and general curiosities.

Regarding viewership levels, there is considerable variation, ranging from over 22 million followers for the most accessed channel on YouTube to 33,000 for the least accessed on X (formerly Twitter), indicating diverse levels of audience accessibility and interest. YouTube hosts longer video content, while X is dominated by text posts with character limits and short videos. Instagram, with over 10 million followers across the top 10 most accessed channels, reinforces its status as one of the leading platforms for disseminating content through integrative tools.

The survey included profiles of professionals, particularly nutritionists, who have large followings on social media. For example, one nutritionist has more than 3.71 million followers. This information is represented in the quantitative data in **Table 1**. The analyzed videos addressed topics such as "How to Relieve Menopause Symptoms?" and offered various natural strategies, including herbal teas, phytoestrogen-rich foods, supplements, and complementary practices such as meditation and vitamin consumption.

The main herbal resources and/or medicinal plants recommended in the posts included *Morus nigra* (black mulberry), *Curcuma longa* (turmeric), *Lepidium meyenii* (Peruvian maca), *Trigonella foenum-graecum* (fenugreek), and, recurrently, compounds such as evening primrose oil and cannabidiol. Frequent mentions were also made of calming herbal teas (such as chamomile, lemongrass, and lemon balm) for managing anxiety and insomnia, as well as foods rich in isoflavones like soy, chickpeas, and lentils, as shown in **Table 1**.

Social network	Views/Followers	Professions	Official website suggested	Period
YouTube	9 channels with approximately 22 million followers	Nutritionists, gynecologists, gastroenterologists	N/A	November 19, 2024 to March 1, 2025
Instagram	10 channels with approximately 10 million followers	Nutritionists, physical educators, gynecologists	N/A	
X (formerly Twitter)	3 pages with approximately 100,000 followers	Nutritionists	1	

Table 1.
Overview of digital social network channels analyzed, including the number of followers, the professional backgrounds of content creators, references to official websites, and the data collection period.

In addition to the quantitative study, a qualitative analysis revealed significant discrepancies between the most frequently cited herbal medicines on social media. Cross-referencing this information with the guideline for the Care of Women in Menopause revealed that only some of these plants have official recommendations, as shown in **Table 2**. The guideline recognizes soy (*Glycine max*), red clover (*Trifolium pratense*), and black cohosh (*Cimicifuga racemosa*) as herbal medicines for managing climacteric symptoms. All these plants have clear technical specifications. For example, red clover (*Trifolium pratense*) requires standardized extracts to guarantee the presence of isoflavones at specific concentrations to ensure clinical efficacy. Black cohosh (*Cimicifuga racemosa*) is also recognized as a herbal medicine for managing menopausal symptoms. It has clear technical specifications, such as the need for standardized extracts that guarantee the presence of isoflavones in specific concentrations to ensure clinical efficacy. There are also contraindications and possible side effects [3].

Social network	Most frequently cited herbal medicines listed in the guideline	Most frequently cited herbal medicines not listed in the guideline	Herbal medicines listed in the guideline but not mentioned
YouTube	Soybean (*Glycine max* L. Merr.), Red clover (*Trifolium pratense* L.)	Fenugreek (*Trigonella foenum-graecum* L.), Blackberry leaf tea (*Morus nigra* L.), Turmeric (*Curcuma longa* L.), Blood orange (*Citrus sinensis*), Flaxseed (*Linum usitatissimum* L.).	St. John's Wort (*Hypericum perforatum* L.) and Lemon Balm (*Melissa officinalis* L.)
Instagram	Black cohosh (*Cimicifuga racemosa* L. Nutt.)	Pumpkin seed (*Cucurbita pepo* L.), Peruvian maca (*Lepidium meyenii* Walp), blackberry leaf tea (*Morus nigra* L.), hibiscus tea (*Hibiscus* spp.), fenugreek (*Trigonella foenum-graecum* L.).	
X (formerly Twitter)	Valerian (*Valeriana officinalis* L.)	Blackberry leaf tea (*Morus nigra* L.), Brazilian ginseng (*Pfaffia glomerata* Spreng), turmeric (*Curcuma longa* L.), Peruvian maca (*Lepidium meyenii* Walp).	

Table 2.
Medicinal plants mentioned during the research on social media platforms.

In contrast, plants such as *M. nigra*, *C. longa*, *L. meyenii*, and *T. foenum-graecum*, despite being widely promoted on social media, are not included in the Ministry of Health's guidelines for climacteric care. Moreover, to date, no robust clinical trials have confirmed their efficacy in alleviating the vasomotor, psychological, or urogenital symptoms typical of this stage of life [1].

An ethnographic analysis of user comments revealed a significant trend: many individuals reported positive experiences with certain plants, noting improvements in energy levels, libido, anxiety management, and a reduction in hot flashes. However, there were also negative comments, with some users expressing frustration over a lack of effective results or even reporting worsened symptoms, such as insomnia or heightened anxiety. These issues might be linked to the improper use of stimulant substances found in some compounds.

In terms of numbers, 70% of the comments analyzed in the sampled videos were positive, while 30% expressed negative views. This highlights the high expectations people have for natural treatments, as well as the potential risks of self-medication and adopting therapeutic practices without professional guidance.

The data suggest that the search for information about menopause on social media goes beyond an interest in physical symptoms; it reflects a profound lack of support, adequate guidance, and sensitive listening in the healthcare system, especially in primary care services. Many people feel that their suffering is minimized or addressed in an overly medicalized way, without considering the complexity of the menopausal experience. This gap is even wider in the case of groups that already face systemic exclusion, such as transgender and non-binary people, whose reality is rarely addressed in public policies or on digital platforms [5].

As a result, there is a growing trend to equate "natural" with safety, well-being, and self-care. However, this mindset often disregards scientific evidence and official medical recommendations. This can lead to the spread of misinformation, especially when people use herbal remedies without proper understanding of dosages, their sources, or standardized phytochemical content.

Based on these findings, it is possible to infer that the digital environment plays an ambiguous role in the context of the climacteric: while it serves as a space for support and the exchange of personal experiences, it also acts as a channel for disseminating content lacking a technical foundation. The scarcity of scientific references in most analyzed posts reveals not only a breakdown in communication between science and society but also a gap in the training of healthcare professionals. In pursuit of visibility on social media, many of these professionals adopt overly simplified narratives, which contribute to the spread of inaccurate information, directly impacting public health [5].

An important finding from the analysis was the widespread conversation about the medicalization of symptoms experienced during menopause. This conversation often included the unnecessary recommendation of psychotropic medications to address emotional changes such as anxiety, depression, insomnia, and irritability.

One social media influencer with 46,200 followers and 101,000 YouTube views presents himself as an expert doctor and directly recommends the use of anxiolytics and antidepressants as a strategy for coping with symptoms, without any mention of integrative approaches, psychological counseling, or non-pharmacological alternatives. This type of recommendation is particularly problematic in the Brazilian context, where there is a well-established culture of self-medication, driven both by ease of access [20, 21] and by the social belief that these drugs are quick and effective solutions for any psychological distress. According to recent data, Brazil ranks among the top countries in global consumption of anxiolytics and antidepressants, with a particular emphasis on use among women. This reality reflects a systematic practice of medicalizing social suffering, in which emotional, social, and existential distress is often treated as isolated clinical disorders. Instead of addressing these demands in a comprehensive manner, the healthcare system tends to resort to medication solutions that often disregard gender specificities and the subjective dimensions of illness [9].

Furthermore, an analysis of content shared on the X platform revealed a disconcerting finding: even institutional profiles, such as the official channel of the São Paulo City Hall, actively participated in the dissemination of information that was not aligned with Ministry of Health recommendations. In a social media post designed to inform the public about menopause, the City Hall's profile recommended therapeutic approaches, including the use of herbal teas, supplements, and soy-derived foods, showing minimal alignment with the Guideline for Women's Care during the Climacteric [3]. Of particular concern is the absence of any scientific references, articles, or technical documents that could substantiate the guidance provided. This absence is a contributing factor to the phenomenon of institutional misinformation. This phenomenon underscores the pervasive nature of misinformation, which is disseminated not only through the channels of alternative therapists and influencers but also via government channels, which, by their very nature, are expected to serve as reliable sources of evidence-based, up-to-date information. This underscores the pressing need for public policies that bolster scientific literacy among the general population and health administrators alike. Moreover, it highlights the necessity for ongoing refinement of informational content disseminated by official institutions.

The results of this study underscore the pressing need for intervention in two key areas: health education and the development of more effective public policies for scientific communication. The integration of data from social media, official documents, and scientific literature reveals a critical disconnect that demands immediate attention. This disconnect must be addressed not only to promote the informed use of herbal medicines but also to strengthen evidence-based care practices that are culturally sensitive and inclusive.

5. Conclusions

The findings of this research show a significant gap between established scientific knowledge, as outlined in official guidelines like the Guideline for Women's Care during the Climacteric, and the information found on social media about using medicinal plants and herbal medicines to manage climacteric symptoms. This gap is not just a matter of misinformation; it highlights deeper issues within the healthcare system, especially in primary care. Primary care is essential, as it serves as the first point of support, providing attentive listening and qualified guidance for individuals undergoing this life stage.

Research has demonstrated that the extensive distribution of unsubstantiated data, frequently originating from authoritative sources such as the official profile of the São Paulo City Hall on the X platform, has a favorable impact on the proliferation of self-care practices. While these practices may be socially accepted, they often lack safety, effectiveness, or consistency. The analyzed posts frequently lack references and promote recommendations that go against official guidelines. This increases the risk of harmful practices, especially regarding the unregulated use of herbal medicines and natural supplements. Such issues have been acknowledged in the literature because of misinformation online, coupled with weaknesses in Brazil's healthcare system and a prevailing culture of self-medication.

Additionally, the analysis uncovered a strong trend toward medicalization during the climacteric phase, characterized by frequent recommendations of psychotropic drugs to handle emotional symptoms. These recommendations often overlook integrative alternatives, psychosocial support, or educational interventions. This issue is exacerbated by the easy access to these medications in Brazil, whether through simplified prescriptions or online purchasing. This reflects a broader trend of medicalizing emotional distress, which historically affects women's health and has increasingly impacted trans and non-binary individuals, who often remain invisible in healthcare and educational resources.

Author details

Ana Claudia F. Amaral[1]*, Débora de Castro Soares[1], Diogo A. Folly[1], Jefferson R. A. Silva[2] and Elaine Cristina Ferreira Dias[1]*

1 Depto de Produtos Naturais, Farmanguinhos – FIOCRUZ, Laboratório de Plantas Medicinais e Derivados - PN1 e Grupo de Inteligência Estratégica e Divulgação Científica, Manguinhos, Brazil

2 Depto. de Química – UFAM, Laboratório de Cromatografia, Manaus, Brazil

*Address all correspondence to: ana.amaral@fiocruz.br and elaine.dias@fiocruz.br

References

[1] Silva MD, da Silva Silveira MA, Guereschi FM. Uso dos fitoterápicos isoflavona e folhas de amora como tratamento no climatério: Revisão sistemática. Revista Concilium. 2022;**22**(6):107-116

[2] Mohapatra S, Kumar PA, Aggarwal A, Iqubal A, Mirza MA, Iqbal Z. Phytotherapeutic approach for conquering menopausal syndrome and osteoporosis. Phytotherapy Research. 2024;**38**(6):2728–2763

[3] Brasil. Ministério da Saúde. Secretaria de Atenção À Saúde. Departamento de Ações Programáticas Estratégicas. Manual de Atenção À Mulher No Climatério/ Menopausa/Ministério da Saúde, Secretaria de Atenção À Saúde, Departamento de Ações Programáticas Estratégicas. Brasília: Editora do Ministério da Saúde, 2008. 192 p. – (Série A. Normas e Manuais Técnicos) (Série Direitos Sexuais e Direitos Reprodutivos – Caderno, n 9. Available from: https://bvsms.saude ./gov./br//bvs/publicacoes/manual_ atencao_mulher_climaterio.pdf/ [Accessed: 2025-June-15]

[4] Kenda M, Glavač NK, Nagy M, Sollner Dolenc M, Oemonom. Herbal products used in menopause and for gynecological disorders. Molecules. 2021;**26**(24):7421

[5] Ferreira VC, Silva MR, Montovani EH, Colares LG, Ribeiro AA, Stofel NS. Saúde da mulher, gênero, políticas públicas e educação médica: Agravos no contexto de pandemia. Revista Brasileira de Educação Médica. 2020;**44**(Suppl 01): e147

[6] IBGE – Instituto Brasileiro de Geografia E Estatística. Censo Demográfico 2022: Unidades de Conservação: Principais Características Das Pessoas Residentes E Dos Domicílios. por recortes territoriais e grupos populacionais específicos: resultados do universo/IBGE: Rio de Janeiro. IBGE; 2025. p. 375

[7] Araújo Ferreira LH, Fonseca Santos T, da Gama Melo JD. Medicamentos fitoterápicos e o uso de Glycine Max no climatério. Scire Salutis. 2021;**12**(1):25-33

[8] Lira FE, and Lira EA. O poder das plantas na menopausa: uma revisão da literatura sobre fitoterápicos como tratamento coadjuvante. Revista Ibero-Americana de Humanidades, Ciências E Educação. 2024;**10** (7):1970–1981. Available from: https://periodicorease.pro.br/rease/ article/view/14924

[9] Arrais PS, Fernandes ME, Pizzol TD, Ramos LR, Mengue SS, Luiza VL, Tavares NU, Farias MR, Oliveira MA, Bertoldi AD. Prevalence of self-medication in Brazil and associated factors. Revista de Saude Publica. 2016;**50**(13s). DOI: 10.1590/ S1518-8787.2016050006117

[10] Nunes AM "Permita que eu fale, não as minhas cicatrizes" Assistência À Saúde da População LGBTQIA+ Através da História Oral de Vida. 2023. Available from: https://repositorio.ufrn.br/bit streams/6c5a1ff5-5e42-4353-b49a-51327 7e65a7b/download [Accessed: 2025- June]

[11] OECD. "The OECD Truth Quest Survey: Methodology and findings",

OECD Digital Economy Papers, No. 369, OECD Publishing, Paris, 2024

[12] Percepção pública da C&T no Brasil - 2023. Resumo Executivo. Brasília, DF: Centro de Gestão e Estudos Estratégicos, 2024. 30 p. Available from: https://www.cgee.org.br/documents/10195/4686075/CGEE_OCTI_Resumo_Executivo-Perc_Pub_CT_Br_2023.pdf [Accessed: 2025-May]

[13] Davis SR, Baber RJ. Treating menopause—MHT and beyond. Nature Reviews Endocrinology. 2022;**18**(8):490–502

[14] Cagnacci A, Volpe A, Di Carlo C, De Leo V, Bifulco G, Gambacciani M, Alfieri S, Biglia N, Bonaccorsi G, Caruso S, Cicinelli E. Phytotherapy for menopausal symptoms: Recommendations of the Italian menopause society (SIM) and the Italian society of gynaecology for the third age (SIGiTE). Italian Journal of Gynaecology & Obstetrics. 2021;**33**(4):214–223

[15] Altawil H, Klawunn R, Dierks ML, Lander J. Parental COVID-19–related health information practises, sources, evaluations and needs: A qualitative interview study. Health Expectations. 2023;**26**(1):555–565

[16] Fernandes LG, Mescouto KA, Costa LO, Saragiotto BT. Ways public health users interact with online health information: A qualitative study. Health and Technology. 2023;**13**(6):905–913

[17] Oliveira TM. Como enfrentar a desinformação científica? Desafios sociais, políticos e jurídicos intensificados no contexto da pandemia. Liinc Em Revista. 2020;**16**(2): e5374. DOI: 10.18617/liinc.v16i2.5374

[18] Teixeira MA, Júnior RN. Levantamento dos Possíveis Remédios Caseiros Disponíveis na Internet para Tratamento do Coronavírus/Survey of Possible Home Remedies Available on the Internet for Coronavirus Treatment. Saúde Em Foco. 2021;**8**(1):49–62

[19] Kozinets RV. Netnografia: Realizando pesquisa etnográfica online. Penso Editora; 2014 June 1. Available from: https://books.google.com.br/books?hl=pt-BR&lr=&id=edi_AwAAQBAJ&oi=fnd&pg=PA1&dq=KOZINETS,+Robert.+Netnografia:+Realizando+pesquisa+etnogr%C3%A1fica+online.&ots=2IHy1mgeSe&sig=K641roVaHdQW-DGW75l0s1TltjU#v=onepage&q=KOZINETS%2C%20Robert.%20Netnografia%3A%20Realizando%20pesquisa%20etnogr%C3%A1fica%20online.&f=false [Accessed: 2025-May]

[20] Castro HC, Santos DO, and Rodrigues CR. Automedicação: Entendemos o Risco? Infarma-Ciências Farmacêuticas. 2007;**19**(11/12):33–36. https://cff.emnuvens.com.br/infarma/article/view/408

[21] Ascari RA, Ferraz L, Buss E, Rennau LR, Brum ML. Estratégia saúde da família: Automedicação entre os usuários. Uningá Review. 2014;**18**(2) 42–47

Chapter 3

Female Sexual Dysfunction and Urinary Incontinence

Diaa-Eldin Taha, Mohamed Tharwat, Reham Ramadan and Ibrahim Alowidah

Abstract

Urinary incontinence (UI) is the involuntary leakage of urine, significantly affecting individuals' social, occupational, and psychological well-being, particularly in women, with prevalence rates between 15% and 55%. UI is linked to sexual dysfunction, with studies indicating that stress-related urinary incontinence affects 26% of women, and 43% of women with urge urinary incontinence (UUI) experience sexual issues such as diminished libido and dyspareunia. The stigma and shame associated with UI can lead to the avoidance of sexual activity, impacting both the affected individuals and their partners. Research shows that UI negatively influences quality of life across various age groups, with severity and type of incontinence being key factors. Women with UUI report higher anxiety levels compared to those with SUI. Treatment-seeking behavior is often hindered by feelings of shame, and women develop coping strategies to manage their symptoms. Sexual dysfunction in women is common, with factors such as age, diabetes, and chronic diseases contributing to its prevalence. Even though UI has a major effect on sexual wellness, research on female sexual dysfunction is less comprehensive than that on male sexual function. UI is classified into three types: SUI, UUI, and mixed urinary incontinence (MUI). Each type has distinct characteristics and impacts on sexual function. Coital urinary incontinence (CUI) is a specific concern, where involuntary leakage occurs during sexual activity, affecting women's self-esteem and sexual frequency. Treatment options for UI include pelvic floor muscle training (PFMT), surgery, and pharmacological interventions, all of which can improve sexual function. Studies indicate that successful treatment of UI can enhance overall sexual health and quality of life. However, the relationship between UI treatments and sexual function remains complex, with varying outcomes based on the type of intervention and individual patient factors.

Keywords: urinary incontinence, female, sexual dysfunction, sexuality, quality of life

1. Introduction

Involuntary urine leaking is known as urinary incontinence (UI), and it can cause serious problems in social and sanitary contexts. The International Urogynecological

Association and the International Continence Society both state that although UI affects both sexes, it is much more common in women, with estimates ranging from 15% to 55% [1]. It negatively affects social, occupational, domestic, and psychophysical well-being [2], and it also imposes financial costs for treatment [3].

Despite the acknowledgment of pelvic floor dysfunction in clinical guidelines established by various international urology and gynecology organizations, there remains a significant gap in addressing the sexual dysfunctions that often accompany UI [4–6]. This oversight is particularly troubling given the anatomical proximity of the reproductive and urinary systems, which suggests a potential interplay between UI and sexual health [7].

In particular, there have been reports of a detrimental effect of UI on sexual function. According to estimates, this occurs in 26% of women with stress urinary incontinence (SUI) and 43% of women with urge urinary incontinence (UUI) [8].

In particular, women with UI have been documented, irrespective of age, to suffer from dyspareunia, vaginal dryness, diminished libido, educational attainment, or race [9]. Furthermore, coital incontinence is a unique form of sexual dysfunction associated with incontinence. Up to 25% of women who visit a urogynecological clinic may experience this, which can be linked to either orgasm or leakage during penetration [10].

Furthermore, UI might condition the avoidance of sexual activity. Sexual inactivity has been found to rise from 35% to 50% in affected women in comparison to controls, and this appears to be directly related to the severity of incontinence [11, 12].

The negative repercussions of UI extend beyond the affected individuals to their male partners, who may experience decreased satisfaction and increased erectile dysfunction [13].

Despite the established link between UI and sexual dysfunction, the full extent of UI's impact on quality of life (QoL) remains inadequately understood, necessitating further research. Existing studies often employ varying definitions and treatment outcomes, complicating the development of a cohesive understanding of this issue [14].

2. Alteration of quality of life (QoL) in patients with urinary incontinence

Using an electronic questionnaire sent to 1,203 women aged 45–60 who lived in the United States of America, France, Germany, and the United Kingdom, Paul Abrams released a study in 2015 that assessed the impact of UI on the QoL of the female population. He confirmed that interference in everyday life (on daily duties, social activities, and perception of mental health well-being) was positively connected with incontinence grade (number of losses per day). The writers emphasized the connection between the intensity of incontinence and the influence on one's familial life, social life, and ability to visit friends [15]. Since it focused on a younger demographic with busy work, familial lives, and social lives, this effort differs from earlier ones. The findings showed that incontinence is linked to a significant feeling of shame and disgrace [16–18].

It affects people of all ages in terms of their QoL [19], and the kind and severity of incontinence are the primary conditional factors. Low self-esteem and an increased risk of mental illness are linked to all forms of incontinence [16]. Because detrusor contractions in UUI are unpredictable, research indicates that women with higher levels of UUI experienced greater psychological stress and worry than those with SUI. Asoglu [1] confirmed that, compared to women with isolated SUI, those with mixed urinary incontinence (MUI) or UUI were more likely to exhibit anxiety and had lower QoL indices. Claudia Senra's Portuguese population survey produced the same findings [20].

The effect on QoL is reflected in the search for care due to incontinence, and there is a correlation between the patient's age, the degree of their incontinence, and the quest for treatment [21, 22]. It is hypothesized that the high frequency of incontinence and decreased treatment search may be connected to shame related to it [17, 23, 24].

Women from various sociocultural backgrounds experience UI intimacy in similar ways, leading to the development of adaptation strategies such as preventing micturition, identifying public restrooms, dressing appropriately to prevent future urine loss, and limiting activities known to be linked to incontinence. They confirmed on a global scale that women and medical experts did not regard light symptoms as significant. The scientists assessed the stigma, shame, and fear related to incontinence and confirmed that the non-White population experienced a greater sense of guilt and a broader negative perception of UI. In contrast to other women, Muslim and Hispanic religious and cultural perspectives on the illness were more pessimistic [17].

3. Female sexual health and dysfunction

Sexual dysfunction is a common problem in the general population [25]. Women's emotional and mental well-being are impacted by their sexual conduct. Consequently, clinical treatment for FSD is becoming increasingly important [26].

It is believed that one factor contributing to sexual dysfunction is the psychological anxiety of urinating during intercourse [27]. Therefore, FSD is partly due to urine leaking [28], 30–50% of women are affected, and the frequency rises with age [29]. According to a prior study, 57% of middle-aged women reported having frequent urination and sexual dysfunction [30]. Diabetes, chronic illnesses, urologic disorders, and cardiac diseases were important risk factors for female sexual dysfunction [31]. According to prevalence research on female sexual dysfunction, between 39% and 45% of sexually active women experience sexual problems [32–34].

Compared to research on male sexual function, women's sexual function does not receive the same level of scientific attention. There is an undervaluation of the sexual component in connection to female reproductive function, and certain functional studies intended for men are modified for women. There is a significant understanding gap between female sexual function, its disorders, and reproductive function [35].

In the 1960s and 1970s, Masters and Johnson came to the conclusion that sexual response happens in four phases: arousal, plateau, orgasm, and resolution. These phases are linear and consecutive. The sexual response model was modified by Helen Kaplan at the end of the 1970s, who emphasized the importance of sexual desire and divided it into three stages: desire, arousal, and climax [32]. Even if individuals do not think of themselves as such, the application of this concept is deemed insufficient.

Only internationally acknowledged features are present for the assessment of dysfunctions, and this is considered when they are excluded: 1) mental disorders unrelated to sexual function; 2) iatrogenic pharmaceutical treatment or clinical conditions that explain symptoms; 3) severe relationship disruption; 4) partner violence; or 5) additional stressors.

The European Urological Association recommends using the following question forms to assess sexual function in the presence of urinary symptoms: ICIQ-VS (International Consultation on Incontinence Questionnaire-Vaginal Symptoms), PISQ-IR (Pelvic Organ Prolapse/Urinary Incontinence Sexual Questionnaire-IUGA revised), FSFI (Female Sexual Function Index), SFQ (Sexual Function Questionnaire), and SQoL-F (Sexual Quality of Life-Female) [4, 36]. All of them have been used in patients with SUI, UUI, and MUI [4]. FSFI [37], ICIQ-VS [38], and the previous version of PISQ-IR (PISQ-12) [39] have been validated in Portuguese.

UI, including stress, urge, mixed, and coital incontinence, has been demonstrated to have a deleterious effect on female sexual function. Treatments for UI, such as pelvic floor muscle training (PFMT), medications, and surgery, appear to enhance QoL by regaining, at least in part, sexual function [40].

A meta-analysis of seven studies found that the overall IIEF score was considerably raised by TOT surgery (mean difference [MD] = 9.74, $P < 0.00001$), erectile function (MD = 1.49, $P < 0.00001$), sexual desire (MD = 2.08, $P < 0.00001$), intercourse satisfaction (MD = 2.36, $P < 0.00001$), orgasmic function (MD = 0.35, $P = 0.001$), and overall satisfaction (MD = 3.46, $P < 0.00001$). However, improvements in IIEF items may have questionable clinical value, as four points in the IIEF's erectile function category are often recognized as the smallest clinically significant difference. Furthermore, nine studies used the Prolapsed Pelvic Organ/ Urinary Incontinence Sexual Questionnaire to interview patients and indirectly analyze the impact of female SUI surgery on the sexual function of male partners. The findings revealed no significant variations in premature ejaculation (MD = 0.07, $P = 0.54$) or erectile function (MD = 0.08, $P = 0.40$) [41].

4. Urinary incontinence classifications

Female UI in adults is categorized into three categories: a) SUI, which occurs when abdominal pressure rises as a result of coughing, sneezing, laughing, or physical activity; b) urgency urinary incontinence (UUI), which happens concurrently with or just after an urgent need to urinate; c) MUI, which affects patients with both stress and urgency urinary incontinence (not always at the same time) [42, 43].

The most common is solitary SUI (51%), followed by MUI (39%), and finally UUI (about 10%), according to clinician interviews and self-administered inquiry questionnaires. Regarding functional urodynamic examination, there is an increase in the pure SUI prevalence (51–77%) and a reduction in MUI (11–39%), while there is no significant alteration in isolated UUI (10–12%) [44].

4.1 Stress urinary incontinence

SUI happens when the pressure inside the abdomen rises, but there is no prior need to urinate. It is determined by the functional capacity of the urinary sphincter, as well as the ligamentous and muscular structures that support the pelvic floor in women. When these mechanisms malfunction and intraabdominal pressure increases (as when lifting weight, coughing, or sneezing), incontinence occurs [45].

Among the risk factors are obesity, age, pregnancy, and vaginal delivery [46]. Incontinence grading is difficult to accomplish. Fultz [47] studied women with UI and found that 28.8% reported moderate to severe discomfort [47].

A research conducted on 111 women in Turkey found that patients' PISQ-12 scores were considerably lower in patients with urodynamic SUI compared to those with UUI ($p = 0.015$), indicating a higher level of sexual function impairment [1, 48]. Women with SUI tended to be less happy with their sexual lives than those with MUI or overactive bladder (OAB), according to a Swedish cross-sectional research study of 147 sexually active women with UI or OAB [49].

In particular, the SUI group experienced a negative impact on sexual desire and/or sexual satisfaction due to insufficient vaginal lubrication, unsatisfactory partner interactions, difficulty in achieving orgasm, and concerns regarding urination while engaging in sexual intercourse. Other research indicated that some sexual issues are especially associated with SUI rather than other forms of UI, such as coital urinary incontinence (CUI) and dyspareunia [50, 51]. In particular, the latter seems to be associated with urethral dysfunction [52].

4.2 Urgency urinary incontinence

UUI refers to the involuntary loss of urine in response to detrusor activity and is a sign of OAB [53]. Alteration of the reflex mechanism in micturition, reduced innervation of the muscular layer of the bladder, and during bladder filling, acetylcholine is released in the parasympathetic neural plaque, activating the bladder smooth muscle via afferents. This process also involves the activation of urothelial receptors (the mucosal layer that covers the bladder) [54].

According to the findings of a meta-analysis on the epidemiology of UUI published in 2014, the prevalence in female patients ranged from 1% to 14%, rising with age and being closely correlated with the socioeconomic standing of those living in the country under study [55].

OAB is a condition that has a significant influence on QoL in the psychological, social, physical, and sexual domains. It can be attributed to neurological abnormalities or idiopathic causes, with the latter being the more common kind. Urodynamic tests may or may not reveal detrusor hyperactivity in these patients.

The goal of UUI and/or OAB treatment is to ease symptoms, and it involves pharmacological treatment, PFMT, and behavioral therapy. Intradetrusor injections of botulinum toxin, neuromodulation (via sacral modulation or posterior tibial nerve stimulation), and bladder augmentation enterocystoplasty are examples of second-line therapy [14, 56].

Research unequivocally demonstrates that UUI impairs sexual function. OAB spectrum individuals were 4.8 times more likely to experience sexual impairment than asymptomatic women, according to a Korean cross-sectional study that used a structured online survey to examine LUTS and sexual activity in 3,372 premenopausal women [57]. Interestingly, even when compared to patients with SUI, those with UUI have poorer sexual function, especially in terms of sexual activity, orgasmic issues, and dyspareunia [8, 48, 58].

4.3 Mixed urinary incontinence

MUI patients describe incontinence as being accompanied by an elevation in intraabdominal pressure, as well as urine loss prior to or concurrently with urgency, without abdominal effort. Patients report variable proportions of urine loss based on physical activity or urgency [59]. It is important to establish which symptom is the most bothersome [60].

The diagnosis is based on the symptoms and the circumstances in which they occur. Urodynamic examination provides little benefit in diagnosis, as detrusor hyperactivity is observed in only 8% among people with urgency in the MUI setting [59].

Although there are no randomized trials on treatments for this disorder, the more bothersome component should be treated according to guidelines, with a lower success rate than those reported in the treatment of separate SUI and UUI [60].

Unsurprisingly, most research indicates that the burden of MUI on sexual function is worse than that of solitary SUI or UUI [61]. In a Turkish cross-sectional study of 118 sexually active women, MUI patients had lower mean PISQ-12 ratings than isolated SUI and UUI patients [62]. From a qualitative perspective, patients with MUI experience a greater negative influence on sexual function across all FSFI domains compared to SUI, UUI, and continent women in the following areas: desire, arousal, lubrication, orgasm, satisfaction, and pain [63].

4.4 Coital urinary incontinence

CUI is defined as the "complaint of involuntary loss of urine during coitus" [64].

It appears that women rarely willingly confer on the matter of coital incontinence unless asked directly by physicians or through self-compiled questionnaires [50]. As a result, compared to other types of UI, coital incontinence may be more challenging to understand and research.

The low frequency of sexual activity among incontinent women can be attributed to a change in self-esteem and image, which is linked to the fear of urine leakage and malodorous incontinence during coitus [65].

SUI was more prevalent in women who had CUI at penetration. MUI with predominant SUI was more common in women who had CUI during intercourse, and UUI and MUI with a dominating UUI component were more common in women who had CUI at climax. Overall, 53.8% of women experienced CUI: 35% during intercourse, 9% during climax, 48% during penetration, and 8% during all four of these periods [66].

The pathophysiology of coital incontinence is not entirely known due to the paucity of data. It is typically divided into two categories: incontinence at orgasm and incontinence during penetration. While the latter is believed to be more common in women with detrusor overactivity, the former is considered to be more prevalent in females with stress incontinence.

While cesarean delivery was protective, prior hysterectomy was a risk factor for CUI at any time. An indicator of body mass exceeding 25 kg/m^2 and prior unsuccessful anti-UI surgery were linked to CUI during penetration and intercourse. Higher levels of UI were substantially associated with CUI and negatively impacted the frequency and quality of sexual activity, according to the results of the ICS questionnaire [66].

The International Female Coital Incontinence Questionnaire (IFCI-Q) was recently created and validated with the express purpose of assessing the type, prevalence, and severity of CUI, as well as its effect on the quality of sexual activity [67]. The authors discovered that up to 77% of patients refrained from having sex, 57% of patients reported that CUI restricted their ability to have sex, and 67% reported that it negatively interfered with their ability to achieve an orgasm.

In 2017, Gray et al. used the Pelvic Floor Electronic Personal Assessment Questionnaire (ePAQ-PF) to assess 2,312 women before their urogynecology session. In comparison to controls, they discovered that women with CUI significantly avoided sex on their own, avoided sex with their partners, and had a lower quality of sex life because of sexual issues [68]. It's interesting to note that all coital incontinence symptoms significantly improved in a subgroup of individuals who received midurethral sling surgery three months after surgery [68].

As stated by the King's Health Questionnaire, CUI has been demonstrated to have a detrimental impact on overall QoL across all areas except sleep and energy [69].

5. Treatment of urinary incontinence and its effect on sexual function

UI is treated globally by 1) PFMT, 2) surgery, and 3) pharmaceutical treatment. The first line of treatment is typically conservative and involves pelvic floor muscle exercises (PFMT). This suggestion is supported by a significant meta-analysis conducted in 2014 utilizing the Cochrane Database, which found that it was beneficial for all types of female UI [70]. A prospective study that supported the advantages of PFMT for improving the QoL for people with UI was published that same year [71].

5.1 Pelvic floor muscle training (PFMT)

Treatments using electrostimulation, biofeedback, and PFMT are all part of the conservative therapy for SUI (pelvic floor muscle strengthening and retraining) [72–74].

According to the literature, effective SUI treatment can raise a woman's total sexual function scores [75]. After six months of PFMT, Bø et al. showed a significant decrease in concerns related to social life, sex life, and physical activity when compared to controls, using validated instruments, specifically the Bristol Female Lower Urinary Tract Symptoms (B-FLUTS) questionnaire and the Quality of Life Scale (QoLS-N) [76]. Similarly, following a 12-month supervised PFMT program in a group of 70 women, Zahariou et al. showed improvements in all domains and the overall score of the FSFI [77].

Studies show that strengthening the pelvic floor muscles in SUI patients, particularly those with coital incontinence linked to penetration, improves sexual performance [1, 78].

It is anticipated that PFMT, which includes pelvic floor muscle strengthening, endurance, coordination, stretching, and relaxation, may improve urge incontinence and sexual dysfunction [81]. Low-frequency electrical stimulation has been demonstrated in studies to reduce local discomfort, enhance pain, and raise the pain threshold [82]. This clarifies why intravaginal electrical stimulation (IVES) helped patients with dyspareunia and FSD feel less discomfort. Furthermore, a progressive sensitivity to pain was brought on by electrical stimulation [82]. Therefore, patients benefited from sustained advancements in pain management.

Dysfunctional pelvic muscle spasm is a protective response to potentially dangerous circumstances. As a result, pelvic muscle rehabilitation is crucial to the treatment of dysfunction, in addition to psychotherapy. IVES strengthens the muscles of the pelvic floor [82, 83]. In one study, vibration and electrical stimulation both increased the effects on skeletal muscle simultaneously [84]. The systolic force acting on muscle fibers may be enhanced by this electrical stimulation and microvibration. Furthermore, concurrent heat treatment improved blood flow and reduced pelvic congestion-related muscular soreness. By creating synergy, the simultaneous delivery of three stimuli or forms of energy can optimize the therapeutic effect [85].

According to the limited research on how PFMT affects female sexual function in CUI patients, women's sexuality significantly improves as a result of fewer incontinence episodes during sexual activity [77, 86]. Additional therapies for CUI are typically based on urodynamic results and may refer to standard management techniques for either SUI or UUI. Sixty percent of patients who received antimuscarinic medication for CUI during orgasm, with verified detrusor overactivity, experienced symptomatic alleviation [87].

5.2 Electrical stimulation for incontinence

It has been demonstrated that biofeedback physical therapy and electrical stimulation are effective in treating female sexual dysfunction in recent years. Clinical practice has made use of IVES and intravaginal biofeedback (IVBF). When women experience spasms in their pelvic floor muscles linked to urinary symptoms, Emma Bendana et al. assessed IVBF/IVES. IVBF/IVES was administered to 52 women, and 64.5% was the average rate of symptom improvement [81, 88, 89]. In order to assess the FSFI scores and PFM parameters, 32 patients with SUI in Korea also received transcutaneous electrical stimulation for eight sessions once daily, five to six times per week; however, no vaginal penetration electrical stimulation device was utilized [81].

Information regarding sexual function following urethral bulking agents is extremely limited. This surgery is typically reserved for individuals who are "unfit" for other antiincontinence surgical procedures due to numerous comorbidities. Consequently, a number of complicating factors may make it challenging to evaluate sexual function in these women. A randomized study comparing TVT (111 patients) with urethral bulking agents (113 patients), based on the PISQ-12 total scores for the treatment of SUI, revealed comparable improvements in sexual function [90]. After a year, there was no difference between the groups, and postoperative dyspareunia remained the same in both.

5.3 Energy based treatment for incontinence

Stress UI has recently been treated with energy-based therapies. In a group of 37 women with SUI, Desai et al. found that radiofrequency therapy improved both sexual function and stress UI based on FSFI scores [91]. Similarly, Kuszka et al. showed that 59 women with SUI who received Erbium YAG laser treatment had improved PISQ-12 scores [92].

There was no difference between laser therapy and radiofrequency therapy, according to a meta-analysis that included four RCTs and two nonrandomized trials (0.26 [95% CI -0.67 to 1.20] and -0.74 [95% CI -3.78 to 2.30], respectively). Energy equipment did not prove that it improved the SF of women with UI [93].

A total of 40 women with OAB and FSD participated in a recent RCT and were randomly allocated to either of two groups: group 1, which received intravaginal electrical stimulation (IVESG) (n = 20), or group 2, which received a placebo control (CG) (n = 20). During the trial, PFMT was administered to patients in both groups, and the IVESG was electrically stimulated for 10 weeks. This study's goal was to contrast how IVES and PFMT affected women's FSD and OAB. Patients in the IVESG showed improvements in their overall FSFI score and domain scores at the end of the research, particularly in arousal and orgasm. The symptoms of OAB also significantly improved. IVES enhanced orgasm and sexual arousal. Overall, our results align with earlier research on [94].

5.4 Medical treatment for incontinence

The effects of various OAB therapies on sex life are less well-established. Zachariou et al. conducted two nonrandomized studies to assess oral therapy, comparing participants who declined treatment with OAB patients on medication (either 50 mg of mirabegron or 4 mg of extended-release tolterodine) [95, 96]. According to FSFI ratings, pharmaceutical therapy improved sexual function in both studies. The impact of second-line therapies for refractory OAB on female sexual function is also not well documented. Two prospective trials were conducted on an idiopathic population with UUI to assess the effects of intravesical injections of onabotulinum toxin A 100 U [97, 98].

An increase in desire, lubrication, orgasm, satisfaction, discomfort, and overall sexual function was noted by FSFI in a short study of 11 sexually active patients who had sacral neuromodulator implantation for OAB. Remarkably, there was no association between FSFI scores and the alleviation of urogenital symptoms [99].

Even after controlling for demographics, social history, gynecologic history, and significant medical conditions, participants with OAB (OABSS < 3) were 23% more likely to report lower sexual frequency (≤ 11) than those without OAB (OABSS ≥ 3), according to a recent cross-sectional analysis of data from the National Health and Nutrition Examination Survey (OR: 1.23, 95% CI: 1.01–1.49, $P = 0.040$) [100].

5.5 Surgical treatment of incontinence

The goal of surgical treatment is to address the functional inadequacies of the urethra and urinary sphincter (Burch surgery, sub-urethral slings, and injection of submucosal polymers surrounding the sphincter) [4, 45, 74]. The success rate ranges from 51% to 91%, depending on the approach taken, the definition of cure, and each patient's follow-up [101].

The cessation of SUI, especially when it is linked to coital incontinence, is thought to be the mechanism by which antiincontinence surgery enhances sexual function [87, 102]. Comparative studies have found no significant variations in the effects of various procedures on sex life. In a 5-year extension of a multicenter randomized controlled experiment comparing midurethral sling and Burch colposuspension, Ward and Hilton evaluated sex life and found no differences between groups [103].

Likewise, it appears that the impact on sexual function is not affected differently by the type of tape. In particular, research comparing the transobturator (TOT) and retropubic (TVT) techniques shows comparable effects on sexual function [104–106]. Jha et al. assessed 113 women with pure SUI who completed the PISQ-12 both before and six months following surgery and who received either TVT or TOT tapes [104]. Regardless of the surgical technique used (TOT or retropubic), a decrease in coital incontinence episodes was noted, and both the physical and partner-related PISQ-12 scores improved after surgery. According to other research, there were no appreciable variations in sexual function between the retropubic surgical techniques and the TOT when comparing the FSFI or PISQ-12 postoperative scores. This seems to be true for both retropubic and TOT tapes, as well as single-incision slings, suggesting that the positive effects of suburethral tapes on sexual function are most likely unrelated to the kind of sling.

The relationship between the surgical treatment of UUI (via sacral neuromodulation) and sexual function is not well explored; the studies that do exist use small patient samples but generally demonstrate improvements in sexual function as measured by questionnaires [107–109]. A meta-analysis published in 2015 concluded that there is not enough information to draw conclusions about how sacral neuromodulation affects female sexuality [110].

Author details

Diaa-Eldin Taha[1*], Mohamed Tharwat[2], Reham Ramadan[2] and Ibrahim Alowidah[3]

1 Urology Department, Faculty of Medicine, Kafrelsheikh University, Kafrelsheikh, Egypt

2 Egyptian Ministry of Health, Dakahlia, EGYPT

3 Urology Department, King Saud Medical City, Riyadh City, KSA

*Address all correspondence to: drdiaaeldin@med.kfs.edu.eg

References

[1] Asoglu MR, et al. Effects of urinary incontinence subtypes on women's quality of life (including sexual life) and psychosocial state. European Journal of Obstetrics & Gynecology and Reproductive Biology. 2014;**176**:187–190

[2] Kwon BE, et al. Quality of Life of Women with Urinary Incontinence: A Systematic Literature Review. International Neurourology Journal. 2010;**14**:133

[3] Hu TW, et al. Estimated economic costs of overactive bladder in the United States. Urology. 2003;**61**:1123–1128

[4] Burkhard F, et al. EAU Guidelines on Urinary Incontinence **73**. Eur Urol: European Association of Urology; 2016

[5] Committee opinion no. 603: Evaluation of uncomplicated stress urinary incontinence in women before surgical treatment. Obstetrics & Gynecology. 2014;**123**(6): 1403–1407

[6] Gormley EA, et al. Diagnosis and treatment of overactive bladder (non-neurogenic) in adults: AUA/SUFU guideline. Journal of Urology 2012;**188**:2455–2463

[7] Visser E, et al. Impact of urinary incontinence on sexual functioning in community-dwelling older women. The Journal of Sexual Medicine. 2014;**11**:1757–1765

[8] Walters MD, Taylor S, Schoenfeld LS. Psychosexual study of women with detrusor instability. Obstetrics and Gynecology. 1990;**75** (1):22–26

[9] Handa VL, et al. Sexual function among women with urinary incontinence and pelvic organ prolapse. American Journal of Obstetrics and Gynecology. 2004;**191**:751–756

[10] Hilton P. Urinary incontinence during sexual intercourse: A common, but rarely volunteered, symptom. BJOG. BJOG: An International Journal of Obstetrics & Gynaecology. 1988;**95** (4):377–381

[11] Coyne KS, et al. The impact of OAB on sexual health in men and women: Results from EpiLUTS. The Journal of Sexual Medicine. 2011;**8**:1603–1615

[12] Brubaker L, et al. The impact of stress incontinence surgery on female sexual function. American Journal of Obstetrics and Gynecology. 2009;**200**:562.e1–562.e7

[13] Bekker MD, et al. Sexual experiences of men with incontinent partners. The Journal of Sexual Medicine. 2010;**7**:1877–1882

[14] Mota RL. Female urinary incontinence and sexuality. International Brazilian Journal of Urology. 2017;**43**(1):20–28

[15] Abrams P, Smith AP, Cotterill N. The impact of urinary incontinence on health-related quality of life (HRQoL) in a real-world population of women aged 45-60 years: Results from a survey in France, Germany, the UK and the USA. BJU International. 2015;**115** (1):143–152

[16] Sinclair AJAR, I.n. The Psychosocial Impact of Urinary

Incontinence in Women. Obstet Gynecol. 1987;**70**(3 Pt 1):378–81

[17] Siddiqui NY, et al. Perceptions about female urinary incontinence: A systematic review. International Urogynecology Journal. 2014;**25**:863–871

[18] Mallah F, et al. Effect of urinary incontinence on quality of life among Iranian women. Journal of Family & Reproductive Health. 2014;**8**:13–19

[19] Brazell HD, O'Sullivan DM, Lasala CA. Does the impact of urinary incontinence on quality of life differ based on age?. International Urogynecology Journal. 2013;**24**(12):2077–2080

[20] Senra C, Pereira MG. Quality of life in women with urinary incontinence. Revista da Associação Médica Brasileira. 2015;**61**(2):178–183

[21] Kwon CS, Lee JH. Prevalence, risk factors, quality of life, and health-care seeking behaviors of female urinary incontinence: Results from the 4th Korean National health and nutrition examination survey VI (2007-2009). International Neurourology Journal. 2014;**18**(1):31–36

[22] Sensoy N, et al. Urinary incontinence in women: Prevalence rates, risk factors and impact on quality of life. Pakistan Journal of Medical Sciences. 2013;**29**:818–822

[23] Choi H, et al. Population-based survey on disease insight, quality of life, and health-seeking behavior associated with female urinary incontinence. International Neurourology Journal. 2015;**19**:39–46

[24] Fritel X, et al. The individual determinants of care-seeking among middle-aged women reporting urinary incontinence: Analysis of a 2273-woman cohort. Neurourology and Urodynamics. 2014;**33**:1116–1122

[25] Aalaie B, et al. Biofeedback versus electrical stimulation for sexual dysfunction: A randomized clinical trial. International Urogynecology Journal. 2020;**32**:1195–1203

[26] Wesche R, et al. The association between sexual behavior and affect: Moderating factors in young women. The Journal of Sex Research. 2018;**56**:1058–1069

[27] Milsom I, Gyhagen M. The prevalence of urinary incontinence. Climacteric. 2018;**22**(3):217–222

[28] Burzynski B, et al. How urinary incontinence affects sexual activity in polish women: Results from a cross-sectional study. International Journal of Environmental Research and Public Health. 2022;**19**(21):13818

[29] Kim JI, et al. Female sexual dysfunction as measured by low sexual frequency is associated with lower socioeconomic status: An analysis of the national health and nutrition examination survey (NHANES), 2007-2016. The Journal of Sexual Medicine. 2021;**19**:90–97

[30] Zhang L, et al. Menopausal symptoms among Chinese peri- and postmenopausal women: A large prospective single-center cohort study. Gynecological Endocrinology. 2020;**37**:185–189

[31] Korchia T, et al. Sexual Dysfunction in Schizophrenia. JAMA Psychiatry. 2023;**80**:1110

[32] Latif EZ, Diamond MP. Arriving at the diagnosis of female sexual dysfunction. Fertility and Sterility. 2013;**100**(4):898–904

[33] Frank JE, Mistretta P, Will J. Diagnosis and treatment of female sexual dysfunction. American Family Physician. 2008;**77**(5):635–642

[34] Castagna G, Montorsi F, Salonia A. Sexual and bladder comorbidity in women. Handb Clin Neurol. 2015;**130**:165–176

[35] Garrett D, Tomlin K. Incontinence and sexuality in later life. Nursing Older People. 2015;**27**(6):26–29

[36] Riss P, Kargl J. Quality of life and urinary incontinence in women. Maturitas. 2011;**68**(2):137–142

[37] Thiel Rdo R, et al. [Translation into Portuguese, cross-national adaptation and validation of the female sexual function index]. Revista Brasileira de Ginecologia E Obstetricia : Revista da Federacao Brasileira Das Sociedades de Ginecologia E Obstetricia. 2008;**30**:504–510

[38] Tamanini JT, et al. The Portuguese validation of the international consultation on incontinence questionnaire-vaginal symptoms (ICIQ-VS) for Brazilian women with pelvic organ prolapse. International Urogynecology Journal. 2008;**19**:1385–1391

[39] Santana GW, Aoki T, Auge AP. The Portuguese validation of the short form of the pelvic organ prolapse/urinary incontinence sexual questionnaire (PISQ-12). International Urogynecology Journal. 2012;**23**(1):117–121

[40] Frigerio M, et al. Quality of life, psychological wellbeing, and sexuality in women with urinary incontinence-where are we now: A narrative review. Medicina (Kaunas). 2022;**58**(4):525

[41] Wang Z, et al. Low-cost male urogenital simulator for penile implant surgery training: A 3D printing approach. 3D Printing in Medicine. 2025;**11**:1

[42] Abrams P, et al. The standardisation of terminology in lower urinary tract function: Report from the standardisation sub-committee of the international continence society. Urology. 2003;**61**:37–49

[43] Legendre G, et al. Menopause, hormone treatment and urinary incontinence at midlife. Maturitas. 2013;**74**:26–30

[44] Correia S, et al. Prevalence, treatment and known risk factors of urinary incontinence and overactive bladder in the non-institutionalized Portuguese population. International Urogynecology Journal. 2009;**20**:1481–1489

[45] Fatton B, de Tayrac R, Costa P. Stress urinary incontinence and LUTS in women–effects on sexual function. Nature Reviews Urology. 2014;**11**(10):565–578

[46] Fallon B, Dwyer NT, Banish S. Stress urinary incontinence in women. Urology. 2006;**13**(Part 1):1

[47] Fultz NH, et al. Burden of stress urinary incontinence for community-dwelling women. American Journal of Obstetrics and Gynecology. 2003;**189**:1275–1282

[48] Duralde ER, Rowen TS. Urinary incontinence and associated female sexual dysfunction. Sexual Medicine Reviews. 2017;**5**(4):470–485

[49] Nilsson M, et al. How do urinary incontinence and urgency affect women's sexual life?. Acta Obstetricia Et Gynecologica Scandinavica. 2011;**90**:621–628

[50] Moran PA, Dwyer PL, Ziccone SP. Urinary leakage during coitus in women. Journal of Obstetrics and Gynaecology. 1999;**19**(3):286–288

[51] Oh SJ, et al. Health related quality of life and sexual function in women with stress urinary incontinence and overactive bladder. International Journal of Urology. 2008;**15**:62–67

[52] Lau HH, Huang WC, Su TH. Urinary leakage during sexual intercourse among women with incontinence: Incidence and risk factors. PLoS One. 2017;**12**(5):e0177075

[53] Haylen BT, et al. An international urogynecological association (IUGA)/ International Continence Society (ICS) joint report on the terminology for female pelvic floor dysfunction. International Urogynecology Journal. 2009;**21**:5–26

[54] Wein A. What are the barriers and how do we manage them? A review of progress over the last 10 years. Canadian Urological Association Journal. 2013;7(9-10 Suppl 4):S172–3

[55] Milsom I, et al. Global prevalence and economic burden of urgency urinary incontinence: A systematic review. European Urology. 2014;**65**:79–95

[56] Barba M, et al. Learning curve of botulinum toxin bladder injection for the treatment of refractory overactive bladder. International Journal of Women's Health. 2022;**14**:1–7

[57] Kim YH, Seo JT, Yoon H. The effect of overactive bladder syndrome on the sexual quality of life in Korean young and middle aged women. International Journal of Impotence Research. 2004;**17** (2):158–163

[58] Coyne KS, et al. The impact of overactive bladder, incontinence and other lower urinary tract symptoms on quality of life, work productivity, sexuality and emotional well being in men and women: Results from the EPIC study. BJU International. 2008;**101**:1388–1395

[59] Gomelsky A, Dmochowski RR. Treatment of mixed urinary incontinence. Central European Journal of Urology. 2011;**64**(3):120–126

[60] Myers DL. Female mixed urinary incontinence: A clinical review. Jama. 2014;**311**(19):2007–2014

[61] Lim R, et al. Effect of stress urinary incontinence on the sexual function of couples and the quality of life of patients. Journal of Urology. 2016;**196**:153–158

[62] Coksuer H, et al. Does urinary incontinence subtypes affect sexual function?. European Journal of Obstetrics & Gynecology and Reproductive Biology. 2011;**159**:213–217

[63] Sen I, et al. The impact of urinary incontinence on female sexual function. Advances in Therapy. 2006;**23**:999–1008

[64] Haylen BT, et al. An International Urogynecological Association (IUGA)/ International Continence Society (ICS) joint report on the terminology for female pelvic floor dysfunction. International Urogynecology Journal. 2010;**21**:5–26

[65] Jha S, Ammenbal M, Metwally M. Impact of incontinence surgery on sexual function: A systematic review and meta-analysis. The Journal of Sexual Medicine. 2012;**9** (1):34–43

[66] Illiano E, et al. Coital incontinence in women with urinary incontinence: An international study. The Journal of Sexual Medicine. 2018;**15**:1456–1462

[67] Gubbiotti M, et al. The International Female Coital Incontinence Questionnaire (IFCI-Q): Development, Validation and Reliability Study. The Journal of Sexual Medicine. 2022;**19**:158–163

[68] Gray T, et al. Evaluation of coital incontinence by electronic questionnaire: Prevalence, associations and outcomes in women attending a urogynaecology clinic. International Urogynecology Journal. 2018;**29**:969–978

[69] Grzybowska ME, Wydra DG. Coital incontinence: A factor for deteriorated health-related quality of life and sexual function in women with urodynamic stress urinary incontinence. International Urogynecology Journal. 2017;**28** (5):697–704

[70] Dumoulin C, Hay-Smith EJ, Habée-Séguin GM. Pelvic floor muscle training versus no treatment, or inactive control treatments, for urinary incontinence in women. Cochrane Database Syst Rev. 2014;**5**:Cd005654

[71] Nyström E, et al. ICIQ symptom and quality of life instruments measure clinically relevant improvements in women with stress urinary incontinence. Neurourology and Urodynamics. 2015;**34**:747–751

[72] Grewar H, McLean L. The integrated continence system: A manual therapy approach to the treatment of stress urinary incontinence. Manual Therapy. 2008;**13**(5):375–386

[73] Bernards AT, et al. Dutch guidelines for physiotherapy in patients with stress urinary incontinence: An update. International Urogynecology Journal. 2014;**25**:171–179

[74] Wood LN, Anger JT. Urinary incontinence in women. Bmj. 2014;**349**: g4531

[75] Beji NK, Yalcin O, Erkan HA. The effect of pelvic floor training on sexual function of treated patients. International Urogynecology Journal and Pelvic Floor Dysfunction. 2003;**14** (4):234–238

[76] BØ K, Talseth T, Vinsnes A. Randomized controlled trial on the effect of pelvic floor muscle training on quality of life and sexual problems in genuine stress incontinent women. Acta Obstetricia Et Gynecologica Scandinavica. 2000;**79**(7):598–603

[77] Zahariou AG, Karamouti MV, Papaioannou PD. Pelvic floor muscle training improves sexual function of women with stress urinary incontinence. International Urogynecology Journal. 2008;**19** (3):401–406

[78] Kao HT, et al. Experience of pelvic floor muscle exercises among women in Taiwan: A qualitative study of improvement in urinary incontinence and sexuality. Journal of Clinical Nursing. 2015;**24**:1985–1994

[79] Sacomori C, Cardoso FL. Predictors of improvement in sexual function of women with urinary incontinence after treatment with pelvic floor exercises: A secondary analysis. The Journal of Sexual Medicine. 2015;**12**(3):746–755

[80] Serati M, et al. Benefit of pelvic floor muscle therapy in improving sexual function in women with stress urinary incontinence: A pretest-posttest intervention study. Journal of Sex & Marital Therapy. 2015;**41**:254–261

[81] Hagen S, et al. Effectiveness of pelvic floor muscle training with and without electromyographic biofeedback for urinary incontinence in women: Multicentre randomised controlled trial. BMJ. 2020;**371**:m3719

[82] Lv A, et al. Electrical stimulation plus biofeedback improves urination function, pelvic floor function, and distress after reconstructive surgery: A randomized controlled trial. International Journal of Colorectal Disease. 2023;**38**:226

[83] Blank C, et al. Assessment of uterine activity during IVF by quantitative ultrasound imaging: A pilot study. Reproductive BioMedicine Online. 2020;**41**:1045–1053

[84] Bae S, et al. Effects of low-frequency intravaginal electrical stimulation on female urinary incontinence, quality of life, and urinary symptoms: A pilot study. LUTS: Lower Urinary Tract Symptoms. 2020;**12**:25–32

[85] Nazarpour S, et al. Effects of sex education and kegel exercises on the sexual function of postmenopausal women: A randomized clinical trial. The Journal of Sexual Medicine. 2017;**14**:959–967

[86] Bø K, Talseth T, Vinsnes A. Randomized controlled trial on the effect of pelvic floor muscle training on quality of life and sexual problems in genuine stress incontinent women. Acta Obstetricia Et Gynecologica Scandinavica. 2000;**79**(7):598–603

[87] Serati M, et al. Female urinary incontinence during intercourse: A review on an understudied problem for women's sexuality. The Journal of Sexual Medicine. 2009;**6**:40–48

[88] Alouini S, Memic S, Couillandre A. Pelvic floor muscle training for urinary incontinence with or without biofeedback or electrostimulation in women: A systematic review. International Journal of Environmental Research and Public Health. 2022;**19**(5):2789

[89] Terlikowski R, et al. Transvaginal electrical stimulation with surface-EMG biofeedback in managing stress urinary incontinence in women of premenopausal age: A double-blind, placebo-controlled, randomized clinical trial. International Urogynecology Journal. 2013;**24**:1631–1638

[90] Itkonen Freitas A-M, et al. Quality of life and sexual function after TVT surgery versus Bulkamid injection for primary stress urinary incontinence: 1 year results from a randomized clinical trial. International Urogynecology Journal. 2020;**32**:595–601

[91] Desai SA, Vakil Z, Kroumpouzos G. Transcutaneous temperature-controlled radiofrequency treatment: Improvement in female genital appearance, sexual dysfunction, and stress urinary incontinence. Aesthetic Surgery Journal. 2021;**41**(12):1400–1408

[92] Kuszka A, et al. Erbium:YAG laser treatment of female stress urinary incontinence: Midterm data. International Urogynecology Journal. 2019;**31**:1859–1866

[93] Pavarini N, et al. Sexual function after energy-based treatments of women with urinary incontinence. A systematic review and meta-analysis. International Urogynecology Journal. 2023;**34**:1139–1152

[94] Piao J, et al. Effectiveness of electrical stimulation combined with pelvic floor muscle training on female sexual dysfunction with overactive bladder: A randomized controlled clinical trial. Journal of Personalized Medicine. 2024;**14**:938

[95] Zachariou A, Filiponi M. The effect of extended release tolterodine used for overactive bladder treatment on female sexual function. International Brazilian Journal of Urology. 2017;**43**(4):713–720

[96] Zachariou A, et al. The effect of mirabegron, used for overactive bladder treatment, on female sexual function: A prospective controlled study. BMC Urology. 2018;**18**(1):61

[97] Balzarro M, et al. OnabotulinumtoxinA detrusor injection improves female sexual function in women with overactive bladder wet syndrome. European Journal of Obstetrics & Gynecology and Reproductive Biology. 2018;**225**:228–231

[98] Miotla P, et al. Impact of intravesical onabotulinumtoxinA on sexual function in women with OAB. Neurourology and Urodynamics. 2016;**36**:1564–1569

[99] Pauls RN, et al. Effects of sacral neuromodulation on female sexual function. International Urogynecology Journal 2006;**18**:391–395

[100] Zhang B, et al. Association between overactive bladder and female sexual frequency: A cross-sectional analysis of the national health and nutrition examination survey data. BMC Women's Health. 2025;**25**:84

[101] Barber MD, et al. The impact of stress urinary incontinence on sexual activity in women. Cleveland Clinic Journal of Medicine. 2005;**72**:225–232

[102] Serati M, Salvatore S, Uccella S, Cromi A, Khullar V, Cardozo L, Bolis P, et al. Urinary incontinence at orgasm: Relation to detrusor overactivity and treatment efficacy. European Urology. 2008;**54**:911–917

[103] Ward KL, Hilton P. Tension-free vaginal tape versus colposuspension for primary urodynamic stress incontinence: 5-year follow up. BJOG: An International Journal of Obstetrics & Gynaecology. 2007;**115**(2):226–233

[104] Jha S, et al. Sexual function following surgery for urodynamic stress incontinence. International Urogynecology Journal. 2006;**18**:845–850

[105] Kim DY, Choi JD. Change of sexual function after midurethral sling

procedure for stress urinary incontinence. International Journal of Urology. 2008;**15**(8):716–719

[106] Murphy M, et al. Incontinence-related quality of life and sexual function following the tension-free vaginal tape versus the "inside–out" tension-free vaginal tape obturator. International Urogynecology Journal. 2007;**19**:481–487

[107] Thiagamoorthy G, Srikrishna S, Cardozo L. Sexual function after urinary incontinence surgery. Maturitas. 2015;**81**(2):243–247

[108] Parnell BA, J.f. Jr H, Geller EJ. The effect of sacral neuromodulation on pudendal nerve function and female sexual function. Neurourology and Urodynamics. 2015;**34**(5):456–460

[109] Caremel R, et al. Results of sacral neuromodulation on the urinary and fecal incontinence and sexuality in 20 women suffering from a double incontinence. Progrès En Urologie. 2012;**22**:424–432

[110] Lombardi G, Agrò EF, Popolo GD. Sacral neuromodulation and female sexuality. International Urogynecology Journal. 2015;**26**(12):1751–1757

Chapter 4

Sexual Dysfunction in Polycystic Ovary Syndrome (PCOS): A Biopsychosocial Approach to Assessment and Management

Yusuf Ziya Kizildemir

Abstract

Polycystic ovary syndrome (PCOS) is the most common endocrinopathy among women of reproductive age, with wide-ranging effects on metabolic, psychological, and reproductive health. An important yet often overlooked consequence of this syndrome is sexual dysfunction (SDF). This chapter provides an in-depth examination of the complex relationship between PCOS and SDF within the framework of a holistic biopsychosocial model. The etiology of SDF is explained by the dynamic interaction of biological mechanisms, such as hyperandrogenism and insulin resistance, alongside psychological mediators such as depression, anxiety, poor body image, and low self-esteem, and social factors such as relational challenges due to infertility. These factors create a bidirectional, self-perpetuating vicious cycle that deepens the clinical picture of SDF. The chapter discusses the role of a multidisciplinary team, a comprehensive clinical assessment using standardized scales, and personalized management strategies. Treatment approaches include lifestyle modifications as the foundation, pharmacological interventions whose potential effects on sexual function must be carefully evaluated, and psychotherapy. Ultimately, it is emphasized that SDF is not a secondary complication but a core biopsychosocial manifestation of PCOS, highlighting the importance of routine screening, patient-centered care, and holistic care for clinicians.

Keywords: polycystic ovary syndrome, female sexual dysfunction, biopsychosocial model, body image, quality of life

1. Introduction

1.1 The intersection of polycystic ovary syndrome and sexual health

Polycystic ovary syndrome (PCOS) is defined as the most common endocrinopathy affecting women of reproductive age, with a prevalence ranging from 6% to 20%, depending on the diagnostic criteria used. This syndrome is far more than a simple reproductive disorder; it is a complex condition with metabolic, psychological, and dermatological manifestations, a multifaceted etiology, and a heterogeneous clinical presentation. Beyond the classic symptoms of menstrual irregularities, infertility, hirsutism (excess hair growth), acne, and obesity, women with PCOS also face long-term health risks such as type 2 diabetes, cardiovascular disease, depression, and anxiety. This complex picture has the potential to impact a woman's quality of life, body image, and overall well-being throughout her lifetime [1].

The World Health Organization defines sexual health not merely as the absence of disease or dysfunction but as a state of physical, emotional, mental, and social well-being in relation to sexuality. This definition underscores that sexual health is an integral and positive component of overall health and quality of life. In the context of a chronic condition like PCOS, sexual health is a critical area that is often overlooked, yet it profoundly affects a patient's quality of life, partner relationships, and psychological well-being. The symptoms of PCOS and the psychosocial burden they create can negatively affect every stage of the sexual response cycle [2].

This chapter aims to provide an in-depth examination of the complex, multifaceted, and often bidirectional relationship between PCOS and female sexual dysfunction (SDF), framed within a holistic biopsychosocial model and informed by current evidence-based data. All layers of the topic will be addressed, from pathophysiological mechanisms and psychological mediators to social dynamics and comprehensive treatment strategies. The goal is to offer a comprehensive theoretical framework and a practical guide to the multidisciplinary healthcare team – including gynecologists, endocrinologists, psychiatrists, psychologists, dermatologists, and dietitians – to manage this complex clinical picture.

2. Pathophysiology and clinical presentation of PCOS

2.1 Definition and current diagnostic criteria

PCOS is a heterogeneous endocrine disorder characterized primarily by chronic anovulation or oligo-ovulation and hyperandrogenism, with an etiology that is not yet fully understood. It is believed that a complex interplay of genetic predisposition and environmental factors contributes to the development of the syndrome [3].

The most widely accepted and utilized diagnostic criteria today are the Rotterdam Criteria, established jointly in 2003 by the European Society of Human Reproduction and Embryology (ESHRE) and the American Society for Reproductive Medicine (ASRM). According to these criteria, a diagnosis is made with the presence of at least two of the following three findings, after the exclusion of other etiologies that could present a similar clinical picture (e.g. congenital adrenal hyperplasia, androgen-secreting tumors, Cushing's syndrome, thyroid dysfunction, hyperprolactinemia) [4]:

(1) **Oligo and/or anovulation:** Clinically manifests as menstrual cycles lasting longer than 35 days (oligomenorrhea) or the complete absence of menstruation (amenorrhea).

(2) **Clinical and/or biochemical signs of hyperandrogenism:** Clinical signs include hirsutism (assessed using the modified Ferriman–Gallwey score),

persistent acne, and androgenic alopecia. Biochemical signs include elevated serum levels of androgens, such as total or free testosterone.

(3) **Polycystic ovarian morphology (PCOM) in ultrasound:** Defined by the presence of 20 or more follicles measuring 2–9 mm in diameter in one ovary and/or an ovarian volume greater than 10 cm^3 on transvaginal ultrasound.

The international evidence-based guidelines, first published in 2018 and updated in 2023, are based on the Rotterdam criteria but introduce important nuances to increase diagnostic precision and avoid overdiagnosis, particularly in adolescents. These guidelines recommend against using ultrasound and Anti-Müllerian Hormone (AMH) levels for diagnosis in young women within the first eight years after menarche, as menstrual irregularities can be physiological during this period. The guidelines promote an evidence-based, consistent, and patient-centered approach to PCOS management [5].

2.2 Key pathophysiological mechanisms

The pathogenesis of PCOS involves a complex network of interrelated and self-perpetuating mechanisms.

- **Hyperandrogenism:** This is the cornerstone and most consistent finding of the syndrome. Basically, it involves an excessive production of androgens (testosterone, androstenedione, DHEA-S) from the theca cells of the ovaries and, to a lesser extent, the adrenal glands. This hormonal imbalance arrests follicular development, leading to anovulation, as well as dermatological symptoms such as hirsutism, acne, and alopecia [6].

- **Insulin resistance and hyperinsulinemia:** A significant majority of women with PCOS (60–95%), particularly those who are obese, exhibit insulin resistance (IR) and compensatory hyperinsulinemia, independent of their body mass index (BMI). High circulating insulin levels suppress the liver's production of sex hormone-binding globulin (SHBG). A decrease in SHBG increases the amount of free, biologically active testosterone in circulation. Furthermore, insulin directly stimulates theca cells in the ovaries and the adrenal glands, further driving androgen production. This creates a vicious cycle in which hyperandrogenism and IR exacerbate each other [7].

- **Chronic low-grade inflammation:** A growing body of evidence suggests that PCOS is a state of chronic low-grade systemic inflammation, characterized by elevated levels of pro-inflammatory cytokines (e.g. C-reactive protein (CRP), interleukins). This inflammatory environment is believed to both exacerbate IR and worsen ovarian dysfunction and hyperandrogenism [8].

2.3 The heterogeneous spectrum of clinical signs and symptoms

The clinical spectrum of PCOS is remarkably broad, and not all patients exhibit the same symptoms or severity. This heterogeneity reflects the different phenotypes of the syndrome. The main signs and symptoms can be grouped as follows [9]:

- **Reproductive findings:** Menstrual irregularities (oligomenorrhea, amenorrhea), anovulatory infertility, and an increased risk of pregnancy complications (recurrent miscarriages, gestational diabetes).

- **Dermatological (hyperandrogenic) findings:** Hirsutism (terminal hair growth in androgen-dependent areas such as the face, chest, and abdomen), persistent acne, seborrhea (oily skin), and androgenic alopecia (male-pattern hair loss).

- **Metabolic findings:** Obesity (in approximately 40%–60% of cases, typically abdominal/central), IR, impaired glucose tolerance, type 2 diabetes, dyslipidemia (high triglycerides, low HDL), and an increased risk of metabolic syndrome.

- **Psychological findings:** High rates of depression, anxiety disorders, poor body image, low self-esteem, and eating disorders.

The flexibility of the Rotterdam "two out of three" rule has allowed the identification of at least four main phenotypes with distinct clinical and biochemical features [4]. This heterogeneous structure demonstrates that the pathophysiology of the syndrome cannot be reduced to a single linear pathway and that each patient exhibits a unique biological, metabolic, and psychological profile. This may be a key factor explaining why the prevalence, type, and severity of SDF vary so significantly from one patient to another. For example, in a phenotype dominated by hyperandrogenism and its dermatological signs, psychological factors (body image concerns, low self-esteem) may be the primary drivers of SDF. In contrast, in a phenotype characterized by obesity and metabolic syndrome, the underlying mechanisms of SDF may be more closely related to vascular and neurological impairments. This understanding is critically important, as it steers clinicians away from a "one-size-fits-all" view of PCOS and, consequently, of SDF, guiding them toward a more personalized assessment and management strategy.

3. Epidemiology and phenotype of SDF in PCOS

3.1 Current classification of female SDFs (DSM-5)

To understand SDF in women with PCOS, it is first necessary to be familiar with the current diagnostic framework for SDF. The Diagnostic and Statistical Manual of Mental Disorders, Fifth Edition (DSM-5), has reorganized female SDFs to reflect the overlapping nature of the sexual response cycle, consolidating them into three main categories [10]:

(1) **Female sexual interest/arousal disorder:** This diagnosis combines hypoactive sexual desire disorder and female sexual arousal disorder from the DSM-IV into a single category. It involves a marked reduction or absence of interest in sexual activity, sexual thoughts, and fantasies, along with a diminished or absent subjective arousal response to sexual cues.

(2) **Female orgasmic disorder:** A persistent or recurrent delay in, infrequency of, or absence of orgasm after a sufficient level of sexual arousal. A marked

reduction in the intensity of orgasmic sensations is also considered part of this diagnosis.

(3) **Genito-pelvic pain/penetration disorder:** This diagnosis merges dyspareunia (painful intercourse) and vaginismus (involuntary muscle spasms that interfere with vaginal penetration) from the DSM-IV. It includes one or more of the following symptoms: marked vulvovaginal or pelvic pain during vaginal penetration or attempts at sexual activity; marked fear or anxiety about this pain; and/or marked tensing or tightening of the pelvic floor muscles during attempted vaginal penetration.

For these diagnoses to be made, symptoms must persist for a minimum of six months and cause clinically significant distress to the individual.

3.2 Prevalence of SDF in women with PCOS: Findings from meta-analysis

Evidence in the literature consistently demonstrates that women with PCOS are at a significantly higher risk of SDF compared to the general population. Meta-analyses in this field have quantified the magnitude of this risk. A comprehensive and frequently cited meta-analysis conducted by Loh et al. found that the risk of developing SDF in women with PCOS was approximately 30% higher than in healthy controls without PCOS. This means the odds of having SDF were 1.32 times higher for women with PCOS compared to their healthy peers [11].

However, it is also important to note that there is no complete consensus in the literature. Some studies, such as one conducted by Zhao et al., have not found a statistically significant difference in the prevalence of SDF between women with and without PCOS [12]. Such contradictory findings likely stem from methodological differences between studies, including the use of different assessment scales for SDF (e.g. FSFI, MFSQ, SDS), varying criteria for diagnosing PCOS, the cultural and demographic characteristics of the populations studied, and differences in study design.

3.3 Affected domains of sexual function: A complex picture

Many studies have shown that women with PCOS score lower in the domains of arousal, lubrication, satisfaction, and orgasm compared to controls [11]. A meta-analysis, while not finding a significant difference in total sexual function scores between groups, highlighted that women with PCOS were particularly prone to reporting dyspareunia (painful intercourse) and a lack of sexual satisfaction [11]. Another review noted that the most common dysfunctions were in the areas of desire, orgasm, and arousal [11].

This variability in epidemiological data and affected sexual domains is likely not a random distribution but is closely associated with the underlying PCOS phenotype, which aligns with the heterogeneous nature of PCOS emphasized in Chapter 1. Most existing studies treat PCOS as a single homogeneous group. However, PCOS is an umbrella diagnosis that encompasses different phenotypes with distinct biochemical and clinical features (e.g. hyperandrogenic-dominant, metabolic-dominant, normoandrogenic). Therefore, it is critically important for future research to examine the SDF profiles by stratifying women with PCOS into these phenotypic subgroups. Such an approach would allow us to move from the general question, "Does a woman with PCOS have SDF?" to a more specific and clinically meaningful question: "Which PCOS phenotype is at higher risk for which type of SDF (e.g. a desire disorder or a pain disorder)?" This is a fundamental step toward personalizing screening protocols and developing targeted treatment strategies.

4. The etiopathogenesis of SDF: A biopsychosocial model

The origins of SDF observed in PCOS are too complex to be reduced to a single factor. This condition is best understood through a holistic biopsychosocial model, in which biological, psychological, and social factors are in dynamic interaction. This model reveals that SDF is not a simple consequence of PCOS but is an expression as heterogeneous and multi-layered as the syndrome itself.

4.1 Biological factors and mechanisms

4.1.1 The paradoxical role of hyperandrogenism

When examining the biological underpinnings of SDF in PCOS, hyperandrogenism plays a central yet paradoxical role.

- **Theoretical expectation versus clinical reality:** Androgens, particularly testosterone, are key hormones in the regulation of female sexual desire (libido) [13]. Based on this physiological knowledge, elevated androgen levels in PCOS could theoretically be expected to increase sexual desire. However, clinical observations and research findings often point to the exact opposite. Low sexual desire is one of the most frequently reported sexual complaints among women with PCOS [11]. The explanation for this paradox lies less in the direct hormonal effects of hyperandrogenism and more in its indirect psychosocial consequences.

- **Indirect negative effects:** Visible dermatological symptoms caused by high levels of androgens, such as hirsutism (male-pattern hair growth), persistent acne, and androgenic alopecia (hair loss), can severely damage a woman's body image, perception of femininity, and sexual self-confidence. A woman experiencing changes she perceives as "unwanted" and "masculine" may struggle to see herself as sexually attractive. This can lead to a range of behavioral and emotional responses – from hiding her body from her partner to avoiding sexual intimacy and, ultimately, social isolation – which fundamentally undermine her sexual life. Research supports these dynamics; while most studies do not find a consistent and strong correlation between serum androgen levels and sexual function scores, they reveal a significant correlation between the severity of hirsutism, poor body image, and SDF [14].

4.1.2 The impact of IR, obesity, and metabolic syndrome

The metabolic components of PCOS constitute powerful and direct biological risk factors for SDF.

- **Vascular and neurological mechanisms:** IR and obesity, which are highly prevalent in women with PCOS, set the stage for SDF through pathophysiological processes similar to those seen in type 2 diabetes. Chronic hyperglycemia and hyperinsulinemia lead to endothelial dysfunction in the small blood vessels that supply the genital area. Endothelial dysfunction alters vasodilation by reducing the bioavailability of nitric oxide (NO). Concurrently, these metabolic disturbances can cause damage to the autonomic nervous system (neuropathy) [15].

- **Consequences for the sexual response:** The physiological basis for female sexual arousal is vasocongestion, the process by which increased blood flow engorges the erectile tissues of the clitoris and vagina. Endothelial dysfunction and neuropathy disrupt this vasocongestive response. Consequently, women may experience difficulty with arousal, insufficient lubrication, and, as a result, painful intercourse (dyspareunia) and difficulty reaching orgasm. Obesity itself can also contribute to SDF by causing physical discomfort and limiting mobility during sexual activity [16].

4.2 Psychological and psychiatric mediators

Although biological factors lay the foundation, psychological and psychiatric conditions play a key mediating role in the onset and perpetuation of SDF.

- **Depression and anxiety:** A diagnosis of PCOS is considered an independent risk factor for depression and anxiety disorders. The prevalence of these disorders is significantly higher in women with PCOS compared to the general population. Depression is inherently characterized by anhedonia (the inability to feel pleasure) and a loss of motivation, which directly suppresses all phases of the sexual response cycle, especially sexual desire. Anxiety, particularly through its cognitive components, such as performance anxiety, fear of rejection, or worry about having a panic attack during sex, can lead to sexual avoidance and arousal problems [17].

- **Body image, self-esteem, and sexual self-confidence:** The visible symptoms of PCOS – weight gain, hirsutism, and acne – can fundamentally disrupt a woman's perception of her body. This leads to body dissatisfaction and feelings of being "unattractive," "flawed," or "masculine." Poor body image directly impacts self-esteem and sexual self-confidence. Negative body perception and low self-esteem are among the strongest psychological predictors of SDF. A woman who dislikes or feels ashamed of her body will find it extremely difficult to open up sexually to a partner, be spontaneous, and focus on the pleasure of the moment [11].

4.3 Social and relational factors

Sexuality is both an individual experience and one that occurs within a social and relational context. The social and relational repercussions of PCOS can further deepen SDF.

- **The role of infertility and menstrual irregularities:** In many cultures, regular menstrual cycles and fertility are seen as core components of womanhood and feminine identity. Chronic menstrual irregularities and the threat or reality of infertility caused by PCOS can fundamentally shake a woman's "sense of womanhood." This may lead her to feel "defective," "broken," or "not a real woman." The process of being diagnosed with and treated for infertility is, in itself, a source of intense stress, anxiety, and despair. During this time, sexuality can transform from a means of sharing love, pleasure, and intimacy into a timed, mechanical, and performance-oriented "task" aimed at achieving pregnancy. This "performance-based sex" destroys spontaneity and pleasure, eradicating sexual desire and satisfaction [18].

- **Relationship dynamics and social stigma:** Infertility can cause tension, mutual blame, disappointment, and communication problems between partners. The partner's attitude – whether supportive or critical – plays a decisive role in the woman's sexual functioning. In addition, visible symptoms such as hirsutism or "hidden" problems such as infertility can cause a woman to withdraw from her social circles (friends, family), fear being stigmatized, and become socially isolated. This isolation reinforces depressive feelings and further harms sexual health [18].

In conclusion, the etiopathogenesis of SDF in PCOS cannot be explained by a simple unidirectional chain of causation. Instead, it involves a biopsychosocial vicious cycle in which each component feeds into and intensifies the others. A biological syndrome (PCOS) leads to a psychosocial crisis, which, in turn, impairs sexual health, thus worsening the biological and psychological state. SDF is not merely a "complication" of PCOS; it is a core biopsychosocial manifestation that lies at the intersection of the biological, psychological, and social dimensions of the syndrome. Therefore, treatment must not only target hormones or symptoms but address all the links in this cycle.

5. Clinical assessment and diagnostic approach

When a woman with PCOS presents with a complaint of SDF, the assessment process must be comprehensive, systematic, and guided by a multidisciplinary perspective. The multi-layered nature of the problem necessitates a holistic approach that transcends the boundaries of any single specialty.

5.1 The role and importance of the multidisciplinary team

The biopsychosocial nature of PCOS and SDF requires the collaboration of various specialties for effective management. An ideal care model should involve a coordinated team that includes the following specialists, tailored to the patient's individual needs:

- **Gynecologist/reproductive endocrinologist:** Establishes the primary diagnosis of PCOS, assesses hormonal and metabolic status, and plans and manages medical treatments for reproductive issues such as menstrual irregularities and infertility. Investigates organic causes of SDF.

- **Dermatologist:** Manages the clinical manifestations of hyperandrogenism, such as hirsutism, acne, and alopecia – dermatological issues that directly impact the patient's body image and self-esteem.

- **Psychiatrist/clinical psychologist/sex therapist:** Diagnoses and treats psychiatric comorbidities frequently associated with PCOS, such as depression, anxiety, and eating disorders. Provides individual or couples-focused psychotherapy and sexual counseling for issues such as poor body image, low self-esteem, and sexual dysfunction itself.

- **Dietitian:** Designs personalized nutrition plans, a cornerstone of the lifestyle modifications essential for treatment. Creates individualized diet programs to facilitate weight management, enhance insulin sensitivity, and improve metabolic health.

Effective communication and coordination within this team ensure that the patient is treated as a whole person, not as a collection of separate issues, and that all aspects of treatment are seamlessly integrated.

5.2 The comprehensive anamnesis: Taking a sexual, medical, and psychosocial history

The foundation of the assessment is a thorough history taken in a safe, empathetic, and non-judgmental environment. The proactive initiation of a conversation about sexual health by the clinician can open the door for the patient to share her concerns.

- **Sexual history:** Structured models such as PLISSIT (Permission, Limited Information, Specific Suggestions, Intensive Therapy) can facilitate the collection of a sexual history [19]. All domains of the patient's sexual response cycle (desire, arousal, lubrication, orgasm, satisfaction) and the presence of pain should be thoroughly investigated. It is important to determine the onset, duration, frequency, and context of the problems, as well as their severity and the degree of personal distress they cause the patient. Communication with the partner about sex and the general state of the relationship are also crucial components of this history.

- **Medical history:** The age of onset, progression over time, severity, and the patient's perception of her PCOS symptoms (menstrual patterns, hirsutism, acne, weight changes) should be documented. Previous and current treatments (e.g. OCPs, metformin, anti-androgens) and their effects on her sexual life should be explored. Other comorbidities, such as diabetes and hypertension, as well as any other medications used, should also be noted.

- **Psychosocial history:** The patient's current mood, anxiety levels, sleep patterns, and sources of stress should be assessed. Her thoughts and feelings about her body (body image), her overall sense of self-worth (self-esteem), and her perception of her feminine identity should be explored. The experience or fear of infertility, the psychological burden it creates, and its impact on the dynamics of the relationship should be addressed with sensitivity. Inquiring about the patient's social support systems (partner, family, friends) can help in understanding her coping resources.

5.3 Standardized scales in assessment and their clinical application

Using validated and reliable standardized scales to convert subjective complaints into objective measurable data is an indispensable part of evidence-based medical practice. This approach improves the precision of diagnostic assessment and allows for systematic monitoring of the response to treatment. These scales provide the clinician with both a baseline and a means to quantitatively track changes over time.

Table 1 summarizes the key scales that can be used in the sexual and psychosocial assessment of a patient with PCOS.

The combined use of these scales provides clinicians with a practical roadmap, reminding them to view an SDF complaint in a patient with PCOS not as an isolated

Assessment domain	Scale name	Abbreviations	Assessed area	Clinical significance and source
Sexual function	Female Sexual Function Index	FSFI	Desire, arousal, lubrication, orgasm, satisfaction, pain (six domains)	The internationally accepted gold standard for identifying the presence, type, and severity of SDF is a total score below 26.55, which indicates SDF [20]
Psychological status	Beck Depression Inventory	BDI	Severity of depressive symptoms in the past week	Widely used to identify and objectively assess the severity of depression, which has a high prevalence in PCOS [21], this tool plays a crucial role in understanding the psychological impact of the condition
	Beck Anxiety Inventory	BAI	Severity of anxiety symptoms in the past week	Used to determine the level of anxiety associated with PCOS and to identify the need for treatment [21]
Self-esteem	Rosenberg Self-Esteem Scale	RSES	The individual's overall level of self-worth and self-acceptance	A critical tool for measuring the negative impact of PCOS on self-esteem and determining the need for psychosocial intervention is essential [22]
Body image	Body Image Scale	BIS	Satisfaction with various aspects and functions of one's body	Assesses body dissatisfaction caused by hirsutism, acne, and obesity, and its potential relationship with sexual dysfunction (SDF) [22]
Hirsutism	Modified Ferriman-Gallwey Score	mFG	Rating of terminal hair growth (0–4) in nine androgen-dependent body areas	A standard method to objectively assess the severity of clinical hyperandrogenism and monitor response to treatment is described in reference [23]

Table 1.
Key scales used in the sexual and psychosocial assessment of patients with PCOS.

sexual problem but as a piece of a larger biopsychosocial puzzle. For example, instead of focusing solely on the desire subscale of the FSFI for a patient presenting with "low sexual desire," concurrently assessing depression with the BDI, hirsutism severity with the mFG score, and body image with the BIS provides a much richer understanding of the origin of the problem. This makes it clearer whether the root cause of low desire is a biochemical process, depression, or a problem of body image related to hirsutism. This approach enables a shift from symptomatic treatment (merely trying to fix the low desire) to etiological treatment (targeting the root cause of the low desire), making the treatment plan much more accurate and effective.

6. Holistic treatment strategies and treatment modalities

Treatment of SDF in PCOS requires a holistic and personalized approach that reflects its multifactorial etiology. The treatment plan must be centered on the patient's individual symptom profile, psychosocial state, sexual concerns, and life goals, such as the desire for children. Improvement in sexual function often occurs in conjunction with, and as a result of, the management of other clinical and metabolic features of PCOS [23].

6.1 The foundational role of lifestyle modifications

Comprehensive lifestyle modifications – including diet, regular physical activity, and weight management – are the cornerstone and undisputed first-line treatment for PCOS. The impact of this approach on SDF is realized through both biological and psychological mechanisms [24].

- **Mechanism of action:** Even a modest weight loss of 5%–10% of body weight can have profound effects on the core pathophysiology of the syndrome. Weight loss significantly reduces IR, which, in turn, lowers compensatory hyperinsulinemia and consequently ovarian androgen production. This hormonal and metabolic improvement can help regulate the menstrual cycle and restore ovulation. A diet rich in unprocessed foods with a low glycemic index, combined with at least 150 minutes of moderate-intensity aerobic exercise per week, is an evidence-based strategy for achieving these goals [24].

- **Effect on sexual function:** Lifestyle modifications target both the biological and psychological roots of SDF simultaneously. Improved metabolic health and endothelial function can enhance genital blood flow, which is essential for sexual arousal and lubrication. At the same time, weight loss and physical activity positively affect the patient's body image, energy levels, and self-esteem. This psychological improvement increases sexual self-confidence and can reinvigorate sexual desire. Thus, lifestyle interventions are the most holistic and least side-effect-prone strategy to manage SDF.

6.2 The effects of pharmacological treatments on sexual function: A risk-benefit analysis

When lifestyle modifications are insufficient or require additional support, pharmacological treatments are introduced. However, while these medications are effective in controlling PCOS symptoms, they can have complex and sometimes contradictory effects on sexual function. This potential risk–benefit balance must be carefully evaluated when selecting a treatment.

Table 2 summarizes the known positive and negative effects on sexual function of pharmacological agents commonly used in PCOS treatment.

This table highlights a fundamental dilemma in PCOS treatment: medications used to treat physical symptoms such as hirsutism (COCs, anti-androgens), which alleviate the patient's psychological burden, have the potential to improve the psychological causes of SDF (poor body image), while simultaneously risking the worsening of its biological causes (low libido). When a clinician prescribes an anti-androgen for hirsutism, the patient's hair growth may decrease and her self-confidence may rise; yet the same drug could cause her libido to decline. This creates

Drug class	Primary indication	Potential positive efforts on sexual function	Potential negative effects on sexual function	Sources
Combined oral contraceptives (COCs)	Menstrual irregularity, hirsutism, acne	Can reduce anxiety and increase comfort during pregnancy by eliminating the fear of pregnancy. Can improve hirsutism and acne, thereby reducing poor body image and associated sexual inhibition.	Increases sex hormone-binding globulin (SHBG) liver production, lowering circulating free testosterone levels, which may lead to decreased libido (sexual desire) in some women. May directly suppress sexual desire via the central nervous system, depending on the type of progestin.	[25]
Anti-androgens (spironolactone, cyproterone acetate)	Hirsutism, acne	Can provide significant improvement in hirsutism and acne, markedly enhancing the patient's body image, sense of femininity, and sexual self-confidence.	By blocking androgen receptors or suppressing androgen production, they may weaken the physiological basis of libido, leading to a loss of sexual desire. Side effects, such as menstrual irregularities, can affect general well-being.	[25]
Insulin sensitizers (metformin)	Insulin resistance, metabolic syndrome, ovulation induction	Targets the core pathophysiology of the syndrome by improving insulin resistance. May improve endothelial function and enhance genital blood flow, supporting arousal and lubrication. Clinical evidence suggests that it improves overall sexual function in women with PCOS, particularly in the domains of lubrication and pain.	Although there are case reports of decreased libido and erectile dysfunction in men, these effects have not been consistently observed in women. Common gastrointestinal side effects, such as nausea and diarrhea, can indirectly impact general well-being and, consequently, sexual desire.	[26]

Table 2.
Known effects of major drugs used in PCOS treatment on sexual function.

a risk of solving one problem while potentially creating another. Therefore, before initiating pharmacological treatment, it is critical that the clinician openly discuss this potential dilemma with the patient and understand her priorities (e.g. "Is your priority right now an improvement in your appearance or the preservation of your sexual desire?"). This enables a truly patient-centered and shared decision-making process. In this context, agents such as metformin, which have the potential to improve both the metabolic profile and certain domains of sexual function, stand out as a particularly valuable option for specific patient subgroups [25, 26].

6.3 The efficacy of psychotherapy and sexual counseling

Given the strong psychological and relational components of SDF, pharmacological and lifestyle interventions alone are often insufficient. Psychological support and therapy should be integral and fundamental parts of the treatment [27, 28].

- **Cognitive-behavioral therapy (CBT):** Targets the dysfunctional cognitive schemas and negative automatic thoughts common in women with PCOS, such as poor body image ("My body is ugly and repulsive"), low self-esteem ("I am inadequate as a woman"), and sexual performance anxiety ("I will not be able to satisfy my partner"). Challenging these thoughts and replacing them with more realistic alternatives helps reduce the associated sexual avoidance behaviors.

- **Sex therapy:** Uses techniques specifically developed for SDFs. This includes addressing gaps in sexual knowledge, correcting sexual myths (false beliefs), improving sexual communication between partners, and employing behavioral exercises like "sensate focus," which emphasizes non-performance-based sexual experiences. Sex therapy has high success rates, particularly in the management of vaginismus (genito-pelvic pain/penetration disorder), anorgasmia, and desire disorders.

- **Couples therapy:** SDF, and especially infertility, are issues that affect not just the individual but also the relationship. Couples therapy addresses the negative impact of these problems on the relationship, strengthens the joint coping skills of the couple, and fosters empathy and emotional intimacy. It helps restructure both their sexuality and their relationship.

These therapeutic approaches help the patient change not only her symptoms but also the way she lives and finds meaning in them, leading to lasting improvement and an enhanced quality of life.

7. Conclusion and future perspectives

7.1 Synthesis of key findings

The evidence presented throughout this chapter establishes that PCOS is a highly prevalent and complex cause of SDF that profoundly affects the sexual well-being of women. The relationship between PCOS and SDF is too multifaceted to be explained by a single mechanism. It is best understood through a holistic biopsychosocial model, in which biological factors such as hyperandrogenism, IR, and obesity are intertwined with psychological factors such as depression, anxiety, poor body image, and low self-esteem, as well as social factors such as infertility, perceptions of femininity, relationship dynamics, and social stigma.

A crucial point is that the relationship between PCOS and SDF operates not as a one-way street but as a bidirectional, self-perpetuating vicious cycle. A biological syndrome causes a psychosocial crisis that, in turn, disrupts sexual health, further exacerbating the biological and psychological condition. Therefore, SDF should not be viewed as a secondary "complication" of PCOS but rather as a core biopsychosocial manifestation of the syndrome itself.

7.2 Recommendations for clinical practice

In light of the data presented, the following clinical practices are recommended for healthcare professionals caring for women with PCOS:

1. **Routine and proactive screening:** The sexual and psychosocial health of every woman diagnosed with PCOS should be routinely assessed at the time of diagnosis and during follow-up visits. Since sexual health is an area where patients often "don't tell unless asked," it is essential for the clinician to raise the topic proactively and with sensitivity. This assessment should be supported by standardized and validated tools, such as the Female Sexual Function Index (FSFI).

2. **Holistic and patient-centered care:** The treatment plan should be personalized by a multidisciplinary team (gynecologist, endocrinologist, dermatologist, psychologist, dietitian) according to the individual symptoms, priorities, concerns, and life goals of the patient (e.g. desire for children). The potential dual effects (risk-benefit analysis) of pharmacological treatments on sexual function should be transparently discussed with the patient, and decisions should be made collaboratively.

3. **Increasing education and awareness:** Raising awareness among patients and healthcare professionals about the profound impact of PCOS on sexual health is of great importance. This will encourage patients to voice their concerns, reduce stigma, and ensure that sexual health problems are recognized and addressed early.

7.3 Research gaps and directions for future studies

Although significant progress has been made in the field of PCOS and sexual health, many questions remain unanswered and research gaps still need to be filled.

- **Phenotype-specific studies:** Future research should go beyond treating PCOS as a homogeneous group and instead stratify patients into different phenotypes (e.g. hyperandrogenic-dominant, metabolic-dominant, normoandrogenic). This will help us understand which phenotype carries a higher risk for which specific SDF subtype (desire, arousal, pain, etc.).

- **A lifespan perspective:** Current research has focused primarily on women of reproductive age. More longitudinal data are needed on the effects of PCOS on sexual development during adolescence and on sexual life during the postmenopausal period.

- **Long-term monitoring of treatment effects:** There is a strong need for well-designed, prospective, randomized controlled trials that compare the long-term effects of current treatments (COCs, metformin, lifestyle modification, psychotherapy) on sexual function, the durability of these effects, and their efficacy in different phenotypes.

- **Novel pathophysiological targets:** The role of novel pathophysiological targets – such as chronic inflammation, the gut microbiome, neuroendocrine pathways, and epigenetic mechanisms – on SDF, as well as potential new treatment strategies aimed at these targets, should be investigated.

- **Partner and relationship factors:** Couples-focused studies are needed to examine more deeply the role of partner factors, sexual communication, and relationship quality in the assessment and treatment of SDF.

Focusing on these research areas will enable the development of more effective, evidence-based, and personalized strategies to improve the sexual health of women with PCOS, thereby enhancing the quality of life for millions of women suffering from this common yet often-neglected problem.

Conflict of interest

The authors declare no conflicts of interest.

Author details

Yusuf Ziya Kizildemir
Department of Obstetrics and Gynecology, Harran University Faculty of Medicine, Şanlıurfa, Turkey

*Address all correspondence to: yusufziyakizildemir@gmail.com

References

[1] Fahs D, et al. Polycystic ovary syndrome: Pathophysiology and controversies in diagnosis. Diagnostics. 2023;**13**. DOI: 10.3390/diagnostics13091559.

[2] Kölükçü E, et al. Association between female sexual dysfunction and polycystic ovary syndrome. Androloji Bülteni (Andrology Bullettin). 2021;**23**(2):87–96. DOI: 10.24898/tandro.2021.15045.

[3] Zalwade PG, et al. Polycystic ovary syndrome (PCOS): A complex endocrine disorder. International Journal of Pharmaceutical Research and Applications. 2025;**10**:566–574.

[4] Joham A, et al. Polycystic ovary syndrome. The Lancet Diabetes & Endocrinology. 2022;**10**:668–680.

[5] Vale-Fernandes E, et al. Should anti-müllerian hormone be a diagnosis criterion for polycystic ovary syndrome? An in-depth review of pros and cons. European Journal of Endocrinology. 2025;**192**:R29–R43.

[6] Wang K, et al. Androgen excess: A hallmark of polycystic ovary syndrome. Frontiers in Endocrinology. 2023;**14**. DOI: 10.3389/fendo.2023.1273542.

[7] Houston EJ, et al. Reappraising the relationship between hyperinsulinemia and insulin resistance in PCOS. The Journal of Endocrinology. 2025;**265**. DOI: 10.1530/JOE-24-0269.

[8] Deng H, et al. Systematic low-grade chronic inflammation and intrinsic mechanisms in polycystic ovary syndrome. Frontiers in Immunology. 2024;**15**. DOI: 10.3389/fimmu.2024.1470283.

[9] Pingping S, et al. Physiopathology of polycystic ovary syndrome in endocrinology, metabolism and inflammation. Journal of Ovarian Research. 2025;**18**. DOI: 10.1186/s13048-025-01621-6.

[10] Parish SJ, Cottler-Casanova S, Clayton AH, McCabe MP, Coleman E, Reed GM. The evolution of the female sexual disorder/dysfunction definitions, nomenclature, and classifications: A review of DSM, ICSM, ISSWSH, and ICD. Sexual Medicine Reviews. 2021;**9**(1):36–56. DOI: 10.1016/j.sxmr.2020.05.001.

[11] Loh HH, Yee A, Loh HS, *et al.* Sexual dysfunction in polycystic ovary syndrome: A systematic review and meta-analysis. Hormones. 2020;**19**:413–423.

[12] Zhao S, Wang J, Xie Q, Luo L, Zhu Z, Liu Y, Luo J, Zhao Z. Is polycystic ovary syndrome associated with risk of female sexual dysfunction? A systematic review and meta-analysis. Reproductive BioMedicine Online. 2019;**38**(6):979–989. DOI: 10.1016/j.rbmo.2018.11.030.

[13] Fernandes T, Costa-Paiva LH, Pinto-Neto AM. Efficacy of vaginally applied estrogen, testosterone, or polyacrylic acid on sexual function in postmenopausal women: A randomized controlled trial. The Journal of Sexual Medicine. 2014;**11**(5):1262–1270. DOI: 10.1111/jsm.12473.

[14] Rusu L, Piele D, Ilie E, Ionescu G, Marin MI, Rusu MR, Calina ML. The

relationship between body composition, physical activity, self-esteem, and body image in female and male adolescents. Sports (Basel, Switzerland). 2025;**13** (1):11. DOI: 10.3390/sports13010011.

[15] Barber TM, Weickert MO, Hanson P, Franks S. Obesity and polycystic ovary syndrome: Implications for pathogenesis and novel management strategies. Clinical Medicine Insights: Reproductive Health. 2019;**13**. 117955811987404. DOI: 10.1177/1179558119874042.

[16] Saadedine M, Nordhues HC, Faubion SS, Kapoor E, Grach SL. Association between obesity and female sexual dysfunction: A review. Sexual Medicine Reviews. 2023;**12** (2):154–163. DOI: 10.1093/sxmrev/qead047.

[17] Cirban Ekrem E, Kavlak O. Polikistik over sendromunda kanita dayali uygulamalar ve hemşirelik bakimi. Arsiv Kaynak Tarama Dergisi. 2021;**30**(2):119–126.

[18] Nasiri Amiri F, Ramezani TF, Simbar M, Mohammadpour Thamtan RA, Shiva N. Female gender scheme is disturbed by polycystic ovary syndrome: A qualitative study from Iran. Iranian Red Crescent Medical Journal. 2014;**16**(2):e12423. DOI: 10.5812/ircmj.12423.

[19] Khoei EM, Kharaghani R, Shakibazadeh E, Faghihzadeh S, Aghajani N, Korte JE and Esmkhani M. Sexual health outcomes of plissit-based counseling versus grouped sexuality education among iranian women with breast cancer: A randomized clinical trial. Medical & Clinical Research. 2019;**4** (6):557–568. DOI: 10.1080/14681994.2020.1732910

[20] Neijenhuijs KI, Hooghiemstra N, Holtmaat K, Aaronson NK, Groenvold M, Holzner B, Terwee CB, Cuijpers P, Verdonck-de Leeuw IM. The female sexual function index (FSFI)—A systematic review of measurement properties. The Journal of Sexual Medicine. 2019;**16** (5):640–660. DOI: 10.1016/j.jsxm.2019.03.001.

[21] Arslan H, Mergen H, Erdoğmuş Mergen B, Arslan E, et al. Eğitim Fakültesi Öğrencilerinin Depresyon, Anksiyete Ve Benlik Saygisi Puanlarinin Farkli Değişkenler Açisindan Değerlendirilmesi. Medical Sciences 2016;**11**:1–13.

[22] Nazik H, Özdemir F, Nazik E, Arslan S. Polikistik over sendromu olan kadınların beden imajı ve benlik saygısı. Ankara Saglik Bilimleri Dergisi. 2014;**3** (1):1–12. DOI: 10.1501/Asbd_0000000043.

[23] Spritzer PM, Marchesan LB, Santos BR, Hirsutism FTM. Normal androgens and diagnosis of PCOS. Diagnostics (Basel). 2022;**12**(8):1922. DOI: 10.3390/diagnostics12081922.

[24] Shahid R, Mahnoor I-U-H, Awan KA, Iqbal MJ, Munir H, Saeed I. Diet and lifestyle modifications for effective management of polycystic ovarian syndrome (PCOS). Journal of Food Biochemistry. 2022;**46**(7):e14117. DOI: 10.1111/jfbc.14117.

[25] McCartney CR, Marshall JC. Clinical Practice. Polycystic ovary syndrome. New England Journal of Medicine. 2016;**375**:54–64.

[26] Misso ML, Teede HJ. Metformin in women with PCOS, cons. Endocrine. 2015;**48**(2):428–433. DOI: 10.1007/s12020-014-0394-8.

[27] American College of Obstetricians and Gynecologists'. Committee on Practice Bulletins—Gynecology. Female sexual dysfunction: ACOG practice bulletin clinical management guidelines for obstetrician-gynecologists, number 213. Obstetrics & Gynecology. 2019;**134** (1):e1–e18. DOI: 10.1097/AOG.0000000000003324.

[28] Barry JA. Psychological Aspects of Polycystic Ovary Syndrome. In: Homburg R, Zouboulis CSeditors Polycystic Ovary Syndrome: Current and Emerging Concepts. London (UK): Palgrave Macmillan; 2019. p. 245–256. DOI 10.1007/978-3-030-30290-0_13.

Chapter 5

Polycystic Ovary Syndrome: A Therapeutic Challenge

María Fernanda Calderón León, Gabriel León San Miguel, Deborah Denisse Gaibor Santos, Rogger Isaac Chinga Acuña, Juan Carlos Suárez Fernández, Andrea Patricia Chancay Mendoza, César Oswaldo Loor Loor, Viviana Carolina Torres Vélez, Liliana Carolina Torres Vélez and Sonnia Paola Diaz Cepeda

Abstract

It is often a therapeutic challenge to manage polycystic ovary/ovarian syndrome (PCOS), as it is a pathology that affects both the metabolic and endocrine systems, generating problems associated with insulin resistance, obesity, and biopsychosocial problems mainly in adolescents and women in the reproductive stage. It affects between 5% and 18% of women of childbearing age. Its etiology is heterogeneous, and its definitive cause is still unknown. Therefore, treatment will depend on each patient's symptoms and individual preferences. It is a common cause of anovulatory infertility in 75% of cases. The objective of this research was to determine the therapeutic challenges of PCOS, for which we reviewed high-level scientific medical articles published in databases such as PubMed, Cochrane, Latindex, Elsevier, Google Scholar, and Embase, concluding that symbiotic supplementation improves several clinical and laboratory aspects of PCOS, including an improvement in hyperandrogenism and lipid profile. In patients with PCOS resistant to treatment with clomiphene citrate (CC), the addition of human chorionic gonadotropin (HCG) at low doses would be an effective method to improve ovulation and, therefore, fertility. The combination of letrozole and clomiphene is superior to either drug separately for ovulation induction in PCOS. Surgical treatment is an option for patients resistant to medical treatment and is performed by laparoscopic or transvaginal ovarian drilling.

Keywords: polycystic ovary syndrome, primary ovarian failure, ovary, treatment, Sclerocystic Ovarian Degeneration, Sclerocystic Ovaries

1. Introduction

It is often a therapeutic challenge to manage polycystic ovary/ovarian syndrome (PCOS), a pathology that affects both the metabolic and endocrine systems, generating problems associated with insulin resistance, obesity, and biopsychosocial problems mainly in adolescents and women in the reproductive stage. It affects between 5% and 18% of women of childbearing age. Its etiology is heterogeneous, and its definitive cause is still unknown. Therefore, treatment will depend on each patient's symptoms and individual preferences. It is a common cause of anovulatory infertility in 75% of cases [1].

Diagnosis in adolescents is a clinical challenge due to the presence of physiological hormonal changes phenotypically similar to those of PCOS, thus requiring early detection of persistent oligomenorrhea and clinical hyperandrogenism [2].

PCOS has genetic and epigenetic etiologies that vary among different populations and families, and it is also considered a risk factor for the development of complications such as metabolic syndrome, cardiovascular diseases, type 2 diabetes mellitus, insulin resistance, and endometrial cancer [3].

Two-dimensional ultrasound is one of the most sensitive diagnostic tests, which usually reveals a minimum of twelve cysts or ovarian volume greater than 10 mL (**Figures 1** and **2**). It is important to know that more advanced imaging techniques can be used in more confusing cases that can broaden the diagnostic perspective; these tests are known as ultrasound elastography, which has facilitated the evaluation of ovarian fibrosis in patients with PCOS by measuring the ultrasonic elasticity index. A systematic review and meta-analysis by Ruan et al. [4] demonstrated that patients with PCOS have greater ovarian tissue stiffness compared to the healthy control group; however, this type of study still requires further research.

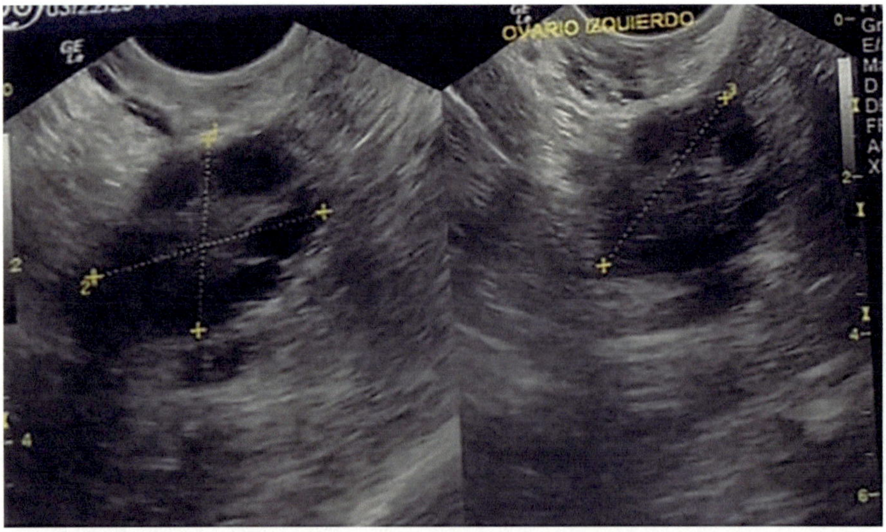

Figure 1.
This image shows multiple oval structures in the form of cysts, located on the ovarian periphery, in a patient with clinical, biochemical, and imaging characteristics of polycystic ovary syndrome.

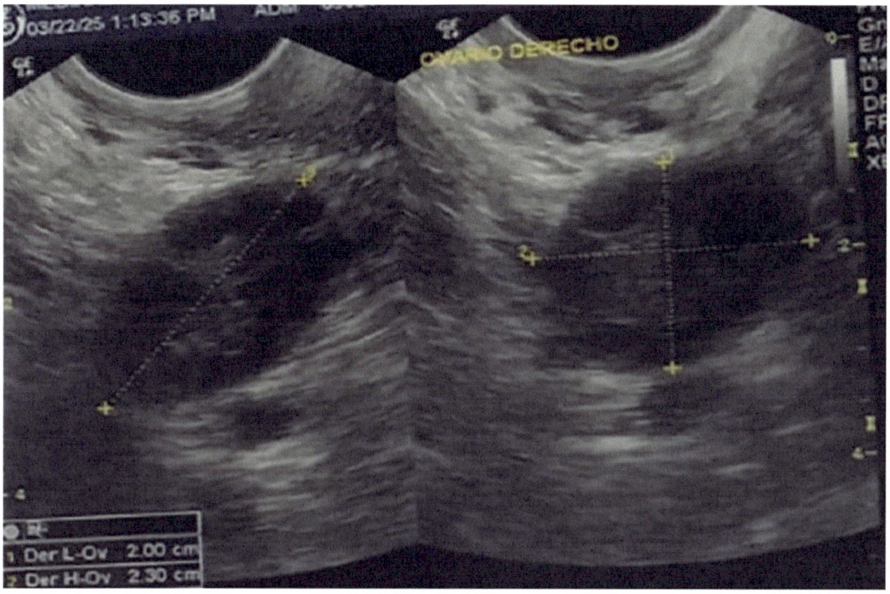

Figure 2.
The presence of multiple cysts located on the periphery of the right ovary of the same patient is evident.

Serum hepcidin could be a potential biomarker for the diagnosis of PCOS, as seen in a study by Nong et al. [5], which showed that serum hepcidin levels in women with PCOS were significantly lower than those of healthy controls. Furthermore, other advances in the diagnosis of PCOS indicate that mitochondrial DNA (mtDNA) mutations have been identified in patients who lack this disorder and are likely to play an important role in its etiology and pathogenesis. It is also important to recognize that, as a chronic low-grade inflammatory disease, patients with PCOS have permanently elevated levels of inflammatory markers (tumor necrosis factor alpha [TNF-α], C-reactive protein [CRP], interleukin 6 [IL-6], IL-8, IL-18) [3].

Patients with PCOS usually visit the clinic with menstrual cycle disorders and are treated with oral contraceptives for hormonal regulation, specifically in relation to follicle-stimulating hormone (FSH) and luteinizing hormone (LH), thus being able to restore the menstrual cycle. However, the effect of hormonal drugs has an impact on metabolic function, mainly on glucose and lipid levels. Therefore, new therapeutic options should be available in addition to general measures to treat PCOS [1].

Exercise and dietary modifications are considered first-line treatments for patients with obesity and PCOS [2]. Numerous studies, such as the one conducted by Turetta et al. [6], highlight the fundamental role of diet in regulating hormonal imbalances that occur in PCOS. Some clinical studies have evaluated the ketogenic diet as a possible benefit for this group of patients [6].

N-acetylcysteine may offer some benefits in the treatment of PCOS but requires a dose adapted to the needs of each patient in order to evaluate its pharmacological effectiveness; however, this drug is still under investigation for its beneficial effects on PCOS [7].

Objective: To determine the therapeutic challenges of PCOS.

2. Methods

High-level scientific medical articles published in databases such as PubMed, Cochrane, Latindex, Elsevier, Google Scholar, and Embase were reviewed. The research question was: What are the therapeutic challenges in PCOS? The search terms used were "polycystic ovary syndrome, ovary, primary ovarian failure, ovary, and treatment." Selected publications that addressed the subject in a clear and precise manner, with results available for analysis.

3. Results

In clinical practice, the treatment of PCOS primarily consists of dietary interventions and exercise, which contribute to a better body mass index (BMI) with weight loss. Secondarily, it can be supplemented with commonly used medications, including oral contraceptives, aromatase inhibitors, estrogen receptor modulators, and insulin sensitizers [8].

In a study conducted by Kataoka et al. (2024), where they evaluated the impact of weight loss on eating behavior, they observed that women with severe obesity and PCOS showed greater cognitive restriction eating behaviors compared to women without PCOS [9].

Several studies, such as the one conducted by Nong et al. [5], have found significant changes in hepcidin levels in patients with PCOS, so it would be important to explore the relationship between PCOS and hepcidin. In a statistical synthesis that included ten studies with 499 cases and 391 controls, the analysis revealed a significant reduction in hepcidin levels in the blood among PCOS patients compared to healthy patients [5].

In a six-month clinical trial conducted by Chudzicka et al. [10] to determine whether the administration of synbiotics affects the endocrine, metabolic, and clinical aspects of PCOS in overweight and obese women who underwent lifestyle modification, the following findings were reported: subjects in the placebo and synbiotic groups experienced significant reductions in BMI and percentage of body fat. However, it is striking that total testosterone was not significantly modified in the placebo group, while it was significantly reduced in the synbiotic group, demonstrating that synbiotics could contribute to the reduction of testosterone in women with PCOS [10].

In a randomized clinical trial involving 300 infertile women with PCOS who were resistant to the effects of clomiphene citrate (CC), researchers evaluated how safe and effective it was to combine the effects of low-dose human chorionic gonadotropin (HCG) with CC to stimulate ovulation in infertile women. They obtained results showing that this combination led to a noticeable increase in the number of ovarian follicles, endometrial thickness, and ovulation rates [11].

In another investigation conducted by Ashkar et al. [12], where they evaluated the therapeutic advantage of the combination of letrozole and CC versus monotherapy in patients with PCOS, a significant effect of the combination of both drugs to induce ovulation was demonstrated and it was concluded that the combination increases the probability of conception and viable pregnancy in women with PCOS [12].

In a study conducted by Foroozanfard et al. [13] on the use of the DASH diet over a period of twelve weeks in women with PCOS compared to the control diet, it showed beneficial effects on anti-Müllerian hormone levels, generating a decrease in the same, as well as a decrease in insulin metabolism, free androgen index, and malondialdehyde (MDA) levels, with significant increases in the quantitative insulin sensitivity verification index, sex hormone-binding globulin, and nitric oxide.

Inositol, also known as myo-inositol (MI) or D-chiro-inositol (DCI), is an organic molecule, formerly known as vitamin B8 that can lower blood glucose and insulin levels by improving the metabolic status of patients with PCOS. Some studies indicate that the dose for this therapeutic effect is 1 g of DCI combined with 400 μg of folic acid per day, improving ovarian function and fertility [14].

A meta-analysis by Roseff and Montenegro [15] evaluated the efficacy of treatments with MI and DCI, alone or in combination, for 12 to 24 weeks and found that nine randomized controlled trials, with 247 cases and 249 controls, showed significant reductions in fasting insulin levels and the HOMA index, demonstrating the efficacy of the therapy.

The abnormal structure of ovarian tissue (fibrosis) is associated with the development of ovarian dysfunction, PCOS, premature ovarian failure, and endometriosis, which affect female fertility and lead to other health problems. Therefore, it is important to further understand the molecular mechanisms leading to ovarian fibrosis in order to develop new treatment methods and thus improve the health of women primarily affected by PCOS [16].

When medical pharmacological treatment has failed, another surgical therapeutic alternative may be applied through ovarian perforation in infertile patients with PCOS. The 2020 Cochrane study compared gonadotropin stimulation and ovarian drilling and found the same pregnancy rate in both cases, concluding that 50% of spontaneous ovulation occurs in the first three months after drilling and 80% of pregnancies occur in the following year [17].

There is a percentage of women with PCOS who have resistance to CC, represented by 15% to 40% of cases, in which ovulation is not observed despite receiving the drug; therefore, a research study investigated the effect of ultrasound-guided transvaginal puncture to induce ovulation. In addition, injectable hormonal medications, such as gonadotropins, can also be offered as a treatment option to induce ovulation in women with clomiphene-resistant PCOS, but it is still unclear, and further studies are needed to determine whether there is a difference between the use of UTND (ultrasound-guided transvaginal ovarian needle drilling) combined with gonadotropins versus gonadotropins alone [18].

In a study with 126 infertile patients, fertility outcomes were compared in two groups of women with PCOS: one group underwent transvaginal ovarian perforation, and another group underwent laparoscopic ovarian perforation, resulting in the finding that transvaginal ovarian perforation is more economical and effective in the surgical induction of ovulation compared to laparoscopic methods [19].

In a randomized clinical study conducted at a tertiary care hospital between June 2016 and December 2018, researchers evaluated the effectiveness of ultrasound-guided transvaginal ovarian puncture to improve fertility in women with PCOS resistant to CC. Twenty-seven infertile women with PCOS were divided into two groups. The first group consisted of patients who received induction with aromatase inhibitors (letrozole 2.5 mg twice daily from Day 2 of the cycle for 5 days) and FSH administered at 75 IU daily from Day 3 of the cycle and maintained until Day 14 of the cycle. Group two received transvaginal ovarian puncture prior to induction with letrozole and gonadotropins, with folliculometry control from Day 9 of the cycle. This group showed significant improvement in serum LH levels, FSH, and testosterone, and also demonstrated an increase in the total number of ovulatory cycles. Pregnancy rates were higher in this study group. The researchers concluded that transvaginal ovarian puncture is a safe and effective procedure [20].

4. Conclusion(s)

Symbiotic supplementation has shown clinical and metabolic improvement, mainly in hyperandrogenism, lipid profile, and endotoxemia markers.

The use of low doses of HCG + CC have been shown to be effective therapeutics for improving fertility in patients with PCOS resistant to CC.

In a good therapeutic alternative, the combined use of letrozole and clomiphene for induction of ovulation in PCOS is effective. Our results conclude that the combination produces improvements in ovulation, cycle characteristics, and secondary changes. Only the incidence of hot flashes as an adverse effect is reported more frequently with the combination.

MI is currently being used with very good results as part of the treatment of PCOS, improving fertility, as is vitamin D, a deficiency of which contributes to the development of PCOS, according to numerous studies.

Surgical treatment is an option for patients resistant to medical treatment and is performed via laparoscopic or transvaginal ovarian drilling.

Expressions of gratitude

We express gratitude toward Lawyer Gladys León Letamendi and Engineer Ángel Calderón Jiménez.

Incompatibility

The authors declare no conflict of interest.

DOI: http://dx.doi.org/10.5772/intechopen.1013041

Author details

María Fernanda Calderón León[1*], Gabriel León San Miguel[2,4], Deborah Denisse Gaibor Santos[3], Rogger Isaac Chinga Acuña[4], Juan Carlos Suárez Fernández[5,7], Andrea Patricia Chancay Mendoza[5], César Oswaldo Loor Loor[6], Viviana Carolina Torres Vélez[1], Liliana Carolina Torres Vélez[1] and Sonnia Paola Diaz Cepeda[4]

1 Catholic University of Santiago de Guayaquil, Guayaquil, Ecuador

2 Scientific Director of Gestar, Guayaquil, Ecuador

3 Catholic University of Santiago de Guayaquil, Guayaquil, Ecuador

4 University of Guayaquil, Guayaquil, Ecuador

5 Technical University of Manabí, Portoviejo, Ecuador

6 Portoviejo General Hospital, IESS, Manabí, Ecuador

7 Technical University of Manabí; Pontifical Catholic University of Ecuador, Portoviejo , Ecuador

*Address all correspondence to: dracalderonleon@hotmail.es

References

[1] Luo P, Li J, Li P, Wang G, Li W, Song Z, Sun X, Fu Z, Zhou H, Yi. A bibliometric and visual analysis of obesity and polycystic ovary syndrome from 2012 to 2022. Frontiers in Endocrinology. 2022;**13**:1011105. DOI: 10.3389/fendo.2022.1011105

[2] Rothenberg SS, Beverley R, Barnard E, Baradaran-Shoraka M, Sanfilippo JS. Polycystic ovary syndrome in adolescents. Best Practice & Research Clinical Obstetrics & Gynaecology. 2018;**48**:103–114. DOI: 10.1016/j.bpobgyn.2017.08.008

[3] Dabravolski SA, Nikiforov NG, Eid AH, Nedosugova LV, Starodubova AV, Popkova TV, Bezsonov EE, Orekhov AN. Mitochondrial dysfunction and chronic inflammation in polycystic ovary syndrome. International Journal of Molecular Sciences. 2021;**22**(8): 3923. DOI: 10.3390/ijms22083923

[4] Ruan Z, Yu Z, Qin Q, Tang Y. Diagnostic value of ultrasound elastography in polycystic ovary syndrome: A systematic review and meta-analysis. Gynecological Endocrinology. 2024;**40**(1):2352139. DOI: 10.1080/09513590.2024.2352139

[5] Nong J, Li H, Yang Y, Lu Q, Sun Y, Yin Q, He H. Low serum hepcidin levels in women with polycystic ovary syndrome: Evidence from a meta-analysis. Gynecological Endocrinology. 2024;**40**(1):2375568. DOI: 10.1080/09513590.2024.2375568

[6] Turetta C, Giannini A, Tarsitano MG, Gianfrilli D, Paoli A, Kontopantelis E, De Angelis E, Minnetti M, Poggiogalle E, Colizza A, De Vincentiis M, Laganà AS, Bogani G, Palaia I, Muzii L, Di Donato V. Impact of the ketogenic diet on weight, metabolic and endocrine parameters in women with polycystic ovary syndrome: A systematic review and meta-analysis. Gynecological and Obstetrical Investigation. 2025;**20**:1–19. DOI: 10.11 59/000543941

[7] Yifu P. A review of the antioxidant N-acetylcysteine in the treatment of polycystic ovary syndrome. Gynecological Endocrinology. 2024;**40**(1):2381498. DOI: 10.1080/ 09513590.2024.2381498

[8] Wu T, Liu Y, Kong F, Hu J, Liu Y, Yang J, Chen J. Improving endocrine and metabolic conditions in patients with polycystic ovary syndrome by acupuncture and its combination therapies: A systematic review and meta-analysis. Annals of Medicine. 2025;**57**(1):2477295. DOI: 10.1080/ 07853890.2025.2477295

[9] Kataoka J, Stener-Victorin E, Schmidt J, Larsson I. A 12-month prospective structured weight loss intervention in severely obese women with polycystic ovary syndrome: Impact of weight loss on eating behavior. Acta Obstetricia Et Gynecologica Scandinavica. 2024;**103**(8):1615–1624. DOI: 10.1111/aogs.14867

[10] Chudzicka-Strugała I, Kubiak A, Banaszewska B, Wysocka E, Zwozdziak B, Siakowska M, Pawelczyk L, Duleba AJ. Six-month randomized, placebo-controlled trial of synbiotic supplementation in women with polycystic ovary syndrome

undergoing lifestyle modification. Archives of Gynecology and Obstetrics. 2025;**311**(2):499–506. DOI: 10.1007/s00404-024-07833-3

[11] Thabet M, Abdelhafez MS, Elshamy MR, Albahlol IA, Fayala E, Wageeh A, El-Zayadi AA, Bahgat NA, Mohammed SM, Mohamed AA, Awad MM, El-Menayyer A, El-Sherbiny M, Elsherbini DMA, Albarakati RG, Alshaikh ABA, Edris FE, Bushaqer NJ, Salama YGM, Abdel-Razik MM. Competition of low-dose human chorionic gonadotropin (HCG) and clomiphene citrate (CC) versus continuous CC during ovulation induction in women with CC-resistant polycystic ovary syndrome: A randomized controlled trial. Medicine (Kaunas). 2024;**60**(8):1300. DOI: 10.3390/medicine60081300

[12] Ashkar A, Jadoon B, Ali Baig MM, Irfan SA, El-Gayar M, Siddiqui FZ. Is the combination of letrozole and clomiphene superior to either monotherapy?: A systematic review and meta-analysis of clinical trials. Gynecological Endocrinology. 2024;**40**(1):2405114. DOI: 10.1080/09513590.2024.2405114

[13] Foroozanfard F, Rafiei H, Samimi M, Gilasi HR, Gorjizadeh R, Heidar Z, Asemi Z. Effects of hypertension diets on weight loss, anti-Müllerian hormone, and metabolic profiles in women with polycystic ovary syndrome: A randomized clinical trial. Clinical Endocrinology. 2017;**87**(1):51–58. DOI: 10.1111/cen.13333

[14] Kamenov Z, Gateva A. Inositols in PCOS. Molecules. 2020;**25**(23):5566. DOI: 10.3390/molecules25235566

[15] Roseff S, Montenegro M. Inositol treatment for PCOS should be scientifically based and not arbitrary. International Journal of Endocrinology. 2020;**2020**:6461254. DOI: 10.1155/2020/6461254

[16] Gu M, Wang Y, Yu Y. Ovarian fibrosis: Molecular mechanisms and potential therapeutic targets. Journal of Ovarian Research. 2024;**17**(1):139. DOI: 10.1186/s13048-024-01448-7

[17] Margaux J, et al. Innovations in ovarian drilling surgery. Journal of Gynecology, Obstetrics and Human Reproduction. 2023;**52**(1):102499. DOI: 10.1016/j.jogoh.2022.102499

[18] Zhang J, Tang L, Kong L, Wu T, Xu L, Pan X, Liu GJ. Ultrasound-guided transvaginal ovarian needle drilling for clomiphene-resistant polycystic ovarian syndrome in subfertile women. The Cochrane Database of Systematic Reviews. 2021;**11**(11):CD008583. DOI: 10.1002/14651858.CD008583.pub3

[19] Hatırnaz Ş, Tan SL, Hatırnaz E, Çelik Ö, Kanat-Pektaş M, Dahan MH. Ultrasound-guided vaginal ovarian puncture compared with laparoscopic ovarian drilling in women with polycystic ovary syndrome. Archives of Gynecology and Obstetrics. 2019;**299**(5):1475–1480. DOI: 10.1007/s00404-019-05067-2

[20] Atwa KA, Farrag MM, El-Sayed MM, Taha OT, Elprince M. Evaluation of the effect of trans-vaginal ovarian needle punctures on women with polycystic ovary syndrome. Journal of Gynecology, Obstetrics and Human Reproduction. 2021;**50**(5):101937. DOI: 10.1016/j.jogoh.2020.101937

Chapter 6

Management of Hypoactive Sexual Desire Disorder

Fabiene Bernardes Castro Vale and Laura de Siqueira Khouri

Abstract

Hypoactive sexual desire disorder (HSDD) is one of the most prevalent female sexual dysfunctions, characterized by a persistent or recurrent lack of sexual fantasies and desire for sexual activity, associated with significant distress and interpersonal difficulties. Affecting up to 15% of women, HSDD remains underreported due to stigma, embarrassment, and limited awareness of treatment options. Its pathophysiology is multifactorial, involving an imbalance between excitatory and inhibitory neurochemical systems, modulated by sex hormones, as well as psychological, relational, and sociocultural determinants. Diagnosis requires both low desire and distress, confirmed through validated tools such as the decreased sexual desire screener and comprehensive evaluation. Management is multimodal, integrating patient validation, sexual education, pharmacological therapies, and psychotherapeutic interventions. Beyond pharmacology, HSDD must be approached as a biopsychosocial phenomenon, with sensitive listening and personalized strategies to restore sexual health and quality of life.

Keywords: hypoactive sexual desire disorder (HSDD), female sexual dysfunction, pharmacological treatment, sex therapy, biopsychosocial approach

1. Introduction

Hypoactive sexual desire disorder (HSDD) is defined as a persistent or recurrent lack of sexual fantasies and desire for sexual activity, associated with significant personal distress and/or interpersonal difficulty, not attributable to a medical or psychiatric condition or the use of substances or medications [1]. Population-based studies indicate that approximately 40% of women report low sexual desire, and approximately 15% meet the primary diagnostic criteria for HSDD (low desire with personal distress) [2, 3]. Despite its substantial impact on health and quality of life, up to 80% of women do not spontaneously raise the complaint with healthcare professionals; more than 50% report discomfort or embarrassment as a barrier to care [3].

2. Pathophysiology of HSDD

HSDD is a multifactorial and complex condition resulting from the interaction among biological, psychological, relational, and sociocultural components. Although traditionally described as a failure of desire, it is now understood as an alteration in the dynamic balance between excitatory and inhibitory systems of sexual desire, modulated by neurotransmitters, hormones, individual experiences, and the interpersonal context [4].

2.1 Biological and neuroendocrine factors

The neurobiology of female sexual arousal involves subcortical and cortical areas that, when exposed to sexually relevant stimuli, can activate or suppress excitatory systems [4, 5]. Sexual response results from the interaction between excitatory and inhibitory neural pathways, mediated by neurotransmitters (dopamine, norepinephrine, serotonin) and neuromodulators such as endogenous opioids (e.g., endorphins), endocannabinoids, and hormone receptors (oxytocin, estrogen, progesterone, androgens, melanocortins) [5].

Excitatory systems: dopamine, norepinephrine, oxytocin, and melanocortins stimulate sexual motivation, reward processing, and responsiveness to erotic stimuli.

Inhibitory systems: serotonin, endocannabinoids, opioids, and GABA act in suppressing arousal, modulating sexual satiety, and establishing the refractory phase.

A predominance of inhibition or a reduction in excitatory activation leads to hypofunction of desire.

During arousal, sexual stimuli activate limbic, hypothalamic, and cortical pathways: Norepinephrine and oxytocin promote arousal, dopamine and melanocortins increase attention and desire, and vasopressin integrates these networks, ensuring a cohesive sexual response. These systems may be stimulated internally by steroid hormones or externally by certain pharmacological agents (**Figure 1**) [5, 6].

Dopamine regulates motivation, reward-seeking behavior, perception of arousal, and hedonic experience. It acts synergistically with oxytocin in the reward system, enhancing bonding, orgasmic response, and sexual desire. Neuroimaging studies demonstrate that dopaminergic circuits are activated during arousal and orgasm, especially in the ventral midbrain. Conversely, dopaminergic antagonists do not alter

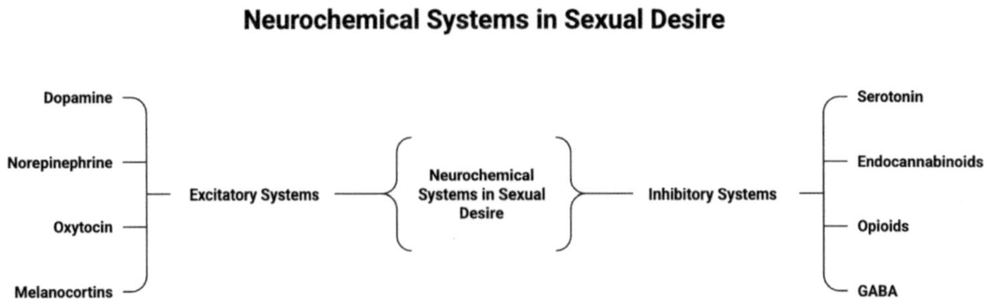

Figure 1.
Neurochemical systems in sexual desire.

learned sexual responses, and dopaminergic agonists do not modify motivation or sexual function in healthy women [5–8].

Sexual inhibition may occur due to physiological refractoriness, natural aversion, or learned avoidance behaviors. In such cases, endogenous opioids and endocannabinoids are released in the limbic system, hypothalamus, midbrain, and cortex, promoting the suppression of arousal and sedation. Serotonin plays a central role in sexual satiety, in reducing motivation, and in controlling reward-seeking behaviors. Elevated serotonergic activity – as seen with SSRIs – reduces motivation and sexual arousal [5, 9].

At the hormonal level, estrogens and progesterone modulate neurotransmission and neural plasticity in hypothalamic and limbic regions. Estradiol promotes oxytocin and α-MSH (melanocortin) secretion, increasing sexual motivation and receptivity, while progesterone is predominantly associated with the suppression of sexual response. Low estradiol levels reduce sexual motivation and contribute to the clinical picture observed in menopausal women with HSDD [5, 10].

Testosterone exerts a stimulatory effect on female sexual response. In the hypothalamus, particularly in the mediobasal region, and in limbic structures, androgen receptors modulate the reactivity of neural pathways to sexual stimuli, inducing arousal. Despite this role, endogenous androgen levels show only a weak association with female sexual desire, with no significant differences in steroid hormone profiles between women with HSDD and age-matched controls [5, 11, 12].

2.2 Psychological factors

Psychological aspects are central determinants in the pathophysiology [4, 12, 13]:

- Mood disorders (depression, anxiety) divert cognitive and affective resources away from eroticism, impairing motivation.

- Chronic stress activates the hypothalamic–pituitary–adrenal axis, increasing cortisol, which suppresses gonadal function and reduces libido.

- Negative body image and low self-esteem impair self-perception as a desiring subject, generating withdrawal and inhibition of sexual engagement.

2.3 Relational and contextual factors

Sexual desire arises in the context of interpersonal interactions [4, 12, 13]:

- Marital conflicts, lack of emotional intimacy, and poor communication reduce sexual interest.

- Lack of privacy and the overload of social roles (work, motherhood, domestic responsibilities) act as practical barriers to sexuality.

- A history of sexual abuse or intimate partner violence is associated with patterns of avoidance and suppression of desire, often reactivated in situations of intimacy.

2.4 Sociocultural factors

Cultural and religious norms that repress female sexuality may generate guilt, fear, or shame regarding erotic expression. At the same time, the media's imposition of unrealistic standards of sexual performance and esthetics fosters body dissatisfaction and insecurity, factors that negatively impact sexual motivation [4, 12, 13].

This complexity explains why HSDD requires an integrated, biopsychosocial diagnostic, and therapeutic approach, considering both the neurobiological mechanisms and the psychosocial and contextual factors that modulate female sexual desire.

3. Recognizing HSDD

The core elements are low desire and clinically significant distress. It is defined as an absence or marked reduction of desire or motivation for sexual activity, manifested by ≥ 1 of the following criteria:

- Reduction/absence of spontaneous desire (thoughts/fantasies);
- Reduction/absence of responsive desire to erotic stimuli; and
- Inability to maintain interest during sexual activity.

The pattern must be persistent or recurrent for ≥ 6 months, occurring with sufficient frequency (though it may fluctuate), and not secondary to a sexual pain disorder or severe relationship problems [1].

Detection is challenging: Many women do not report the complaint spontaneously; physicians often do not initiate the conversation due to limited time, discomfort, or the perception of limited therapeutic options.

4. Engaging the patient: Screening for HSDD

Screening can be brief and structured during consultation, investigating sexual activity, concerns about desire, and satisfaction with the current level. If concerns are identified, formal screening is recommended. A useful tool is the Decreased Sexual Desire Screener (DSDS), a validated instrument consisting of five yes/no items, which assists in distinguishing generalized from situational forms of HSDD, as illustrated in **Figure 2** [14].

A useful tool is the decreased sexual desire screener (DSDS) [14], consisting of five yes/no items:

- YES to Questions 1–4 and NO to all factors in Question 5 → generalized acquired HSDD.
- YES to Questions 1–4 and YES to any factor in Question 5 → situational, acquired HSDD.
- NO to any of Questions 1–4 → does not qualify as HSDD.

Decreased Sexual Desire Screener (DSDS)

Dear Patient,
Please answer each of the following questions:

1. In the past was your level of sexual desire or interest good and satisfying to you? Yes/No
2. Has there been a decrease in your level of sexual desire or interest? Yes/No
3. Are you bothered by your decreased level of sexual desire or interest? Yes/No
4. Would you like your level of sexual desire or interest to increase? Yes/No
5. Please check all the factors that you feel may be contributing to your current decrease in sexual desire or interest: Yes/No
A: An operation, depression, injuries, or other medical condition
B: Medication, drugs or alcohol you are currently taking
C: Pregnancy, recent childbirth, menopausal symptoms
D: Other sexual issues you may be having (pain, decreased arousal or orgasm)
E: Your partner's sexual problems
F: Dissatisfaction with your relationship or partner
G: Stress or fatigue

Figure 2.
Decreased sexual desire screener.

5. Assessment of HSDD

Once suspicion is confirmed, the diagnostic evaluation of HSDD should follow. The assessment must be systematic, integrating clinical, psychological, and relational aspects, with the aim of confirming the presence of the disorder, identifying contributory factors, and establishing the foundation for an individualized therapeutic plan [15].

5.1 General medical history

The medical history should be comprehensive, addressing the following:

- **Organic comorbidities:** endocrine diseases (hypothyroidism, diabetes mellitus, polycystic ovary syndrome), neurological, cardiovascular, or oncological conditions that may affect sexual desire.
- **Surgical and gynecological history:** hysterectomy, oophorectomy, pelvic surgeries, radiotherapy, or chemotherapy.
- **Medication use:** antidepressants (particularly SSRIs and SNRIs), antihypertensives, anticonvulsants, hormonal contraceptives, and other agents capable of influencing neurotransmission or hormone levels.
- **Lifestyle factors:** smoking, alcohol consumption, and illicit drug use.
- **Psychological and social conditions:** chronic stress, role overload, family support.
- **Relational context:** marital satisfaction, presence of conflicts, communication with the partner.

5.2 Detailed sexual history

The sexual interview should be conducted in a safe, welcoming, and nonjudgmental environment, using open-ended questions that allow exploration of the patient's subjectivity:

- **Desire and interest**
  Do you feel interested or have the desire to initiate a sexual relationship? How would you describe your current level of sexual desire?

- **Sexual fantasies**
  Do you usually have sexual thoughts or fantasies?

- **Responsive desire**
  When sexual stimulation occurs (touch, kiss, caress), do you feel inclined to continue with the stimuli or proceed with intercourse?

- **Temporal characterization**
  Differentiate lifelong (present since the beginning of sexual life) from acquired (emerging after a period of normal sexual function).

- **Scope**
  Differentiate generalized (in all contexts/partners) from situational (restricted to specific situations or partners).

- **Triggering factors**
  Explore life events, the onset of medications, hormonal changes, and stressful circumstances.

- **Subjective and interpersonal impact**
  Identify personal distress and relationship difficulties directly associated with low desire.

5.3 Relational assessment and risk factors

- **Relationship quality:** shared interests, quality of communication, and time dedicated to couple leisure.

- **Partner's sexual dysfunctions:** the presence of erectile, ejaculatory, or desire difficulties, which may influence the patient's complaint.

- **History of violence and sexual trauma:** investigated intimate partner violence, traumatic experiences in childhood/adolescence, or sexual coercion, given their strong impact on future sexual function.

5.4 Physical examination and complementary tests

In addition to the medical history, a targeted physical examination is recommended (gynecological examination, assessment of external genitalia, vaginal mucosa, pelvic floor tone) and, when necessary, laboratory tests (hormonal, thyroid, glycemic, lipid profiles) to exclude concomitant organic causes.

Once the clinical criteria for HSDD are confirmed – persistent or recurrent reduction in sexual desire associated with significant personal distress – the diagnosis should be validated with the patient. This moment is essential to legitimize the complaint, reduce feelings of guilt or inadequacy, and introduce the discussion of personalized therapeutic strategies.

6. Treatment of HSDD

The treatment is etiological and multimodal, beginning with validation of the patient's complaint, followed by sexual education, and subsequently combining pharmacological measures (hormonal and nonhormonal) with psychotherapy (sex therapy, CBT) [16].

6.1 Validation of the patient's complaint

A crucial step in caring for women with HSDD is validating the complaint. Sexuality often remains invisible in clinical practice, and the patient may have internalized feelings of guilt, shame, or inadequacy [17]. By acknowledging the suffering as legitimate, the professional:

- normalizes the experience, demonstrating that it is neither isolated nor abnormal;
- reduces the stigma associated with female sexual health; and
- strengthens the therapeutic alliance, creating a safe space for open dialog.

This validation has a direct clinical impact as it increases treatment adherence and motivates the patient to explore strategies for managing sexual desire.

6.2 Sexual education

In sexual education, the first step should be explaining the female sexual response, presented in accessible language but grounded in science [17]. This clarification is essential to deconstruct myths and validate individual experiences, highlighting the two fundamental patterns of desire:

- **Spontaneous desire:** It is characterized by the emergence of fantasies, erotic thoughts, or the urge for sexual activity without an immediate external stimulus. It is more frequent during phases of heightened hormonal activation, at the beginning of relationships, or in contexts of erotic novelty.
- **Responsive desire:** It arises after erotic stimulation or intimate interaction, being awakened during the sexual experience, even if there is no initial intention to initiate intercourse. This model is especially prevalent in women in long-term relationships.

Sexual education must emphasize that both patterns are normal and that the absence of spontaneous desire does not represent failure, but rather a shift in the way desire manifests. Recognizing responsive desire as healthy helps the patient (and her partner) understand that desire can be cultivated and restored through intimacy, communication, and erotic stimulation [17].

6.3 Guidance for restoring desire: The theory of the rupture of the three pillars of communication

Understanding sexual response is only the first step; the second is to provide practical pathways for restoring erotic dynamics in the couple. Restoring sexual desire goes beyond the biological sphere and requires rebuilding intimate communication, understood as a continuous process of affective, emotional, and symbolic exchange [18]. This conceptual framework, illustrating the rupture of the three pillars of communication—indifference, fear, and dependence—and their relationship to the restoration of sexual desire, is depicted in **Figure 3**. In this sense, the theory of the rupture of the three pillars of communication describes dynamics that weaken intimacy and reduce sexual desire:

- **Indifference**

  It is characterized by the erosion of attention, care, and listening in the relationship. The partner becomes neutral, predictable, or emotionally distant, generating in the woman a sense of invisibility and loss of erotic value.

  Therapeutic strategy

  It encourages practices of mutual recognition and appreciation – genuine compliments, demonstrations of interest in daily life, reinforcement of personal achievements, and resumption of affectionate rituals – promoting the rekindling of the bond and the perception of being desired and desiring.

- **Fear**

  It manifests when intimate dialog is permeated by the fear of criticism, rejection, or emotional punishment. The patient may inhibit the expression of fantasies and preferences, establishing an erotic silence that corrodes spontaneity.

  Therapeutic strategy

  It fosters a communicational space that is safe and trust-based, encouraging active listening, empathy, and emotional validation, reinforcing the idea that eroticism flourishes when vulnerability is welcomed and respected.

- **Dependence**

  It occurs when there is an imbalance of power, and one partner conditions their self-esteem or identity on the other's approval. This dynamic imprisons sexuality in a model of submission and passivity, undermining the woman's erotic autonomy.

  Therapeutic strategy

  It strengthens the woman's self-perception as a subject of desire, encouraging practices of self-exploration, self-knowledge, and recovery of individuality while working to rebalance power within the relationship.

  The restoration of the three pillars – attention (antidote to indifference), trust (antidote to fear), and autonomy (antidote to dependence) – is an essential condition for rebuilding sexual desire. This integrative process, progressing from diminished sexual desire to rekindled erotic vitality through the strengthening of attention, trust, and autonomy, is illustrated in **Figure 4**. Thus, sexual education must be multidimensional: In addition to providing scientific knowledge, it should offer practical tools to restore intimate dialog, strengthen affective reciprocity, and rekindle erotic vitality within the couple [17, 18].

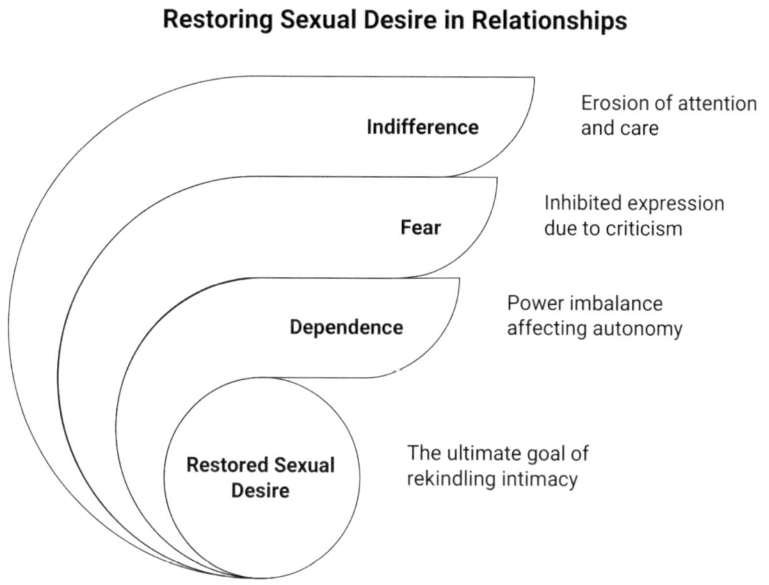

Figure 3.
Restoring sexual desire in relationships.

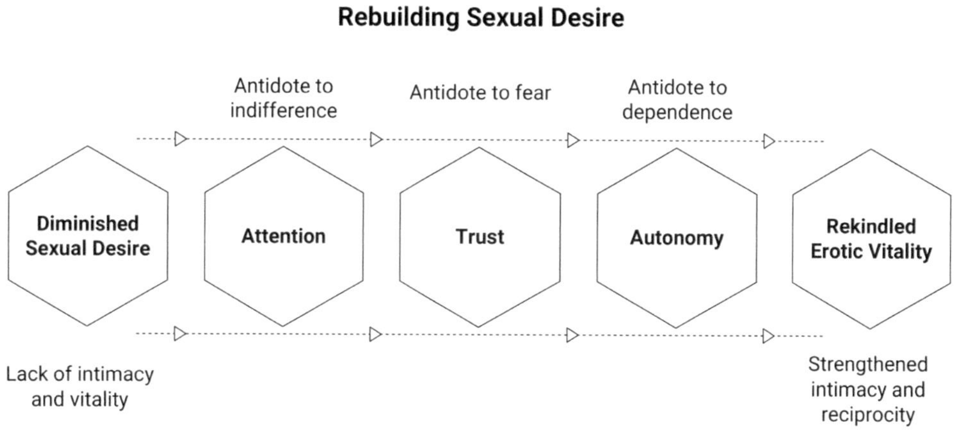

Figure 4.
Rebuilding sexual desire.

6.4 Pharmacological measures

Hormone therapy (HT)

HT can be effective in postmenopausal women with HSDD, especially when hypoestrogenism (vulvovaginal/pelvic floor impact), vasomotor symptoms, and sleep disturbances coexist. Ovarian and adrenal androgen production decline with age, and testosterone levels at age 50 approach approximately 50% of those seen in the 20s. Testosterone contributes to desire activation, arousal, and sensitivity.

In women with climacteric symptoms and reduced libido, HT may be indicated, in the absence of contraindications, with specific agents.

- **Tibolone 2.5 mg PO daily** (synthetic steroid derived from norethisterone, with estrogenic, progestogenic, and androgenic tissue actions): It is indicated in postmenopause within the "window of opportunity" in women with HSDD. *Absolute contraindications*: breast/endometrial cancer, acute thromboembolism, acute/severe hepatopathy, severe cardiopathy, and unexplained uterine bleeding. *Benefits:* increased desire, arousal, frequency, satisfaction, and positive urogenital effect; modulates endorphins and improves well-being/quality of life (evidence level 2) [19].

- **Estrogen therapy (ET):** Although effective for relieving climacteric symptoms, it does not exert a direct and robust effect on desire, arousal, or orgasm. In women with climacteric symptoms and reduced libido under HT, transdermal formulations are preferred (lower SHBG elevation, preserving free testosterone) [20]. *With a uterus*: combine transdermal estrogen with natural progesterone. *Without a uterus*: transdermal ET alone may be an option.

- **Androgen therapy (AT):** no licensed formulations of testosterone for women are available (FDA/ANVISA). 1% creams/gels (≈0.5 g/day) applied to the skin (arms, legs, abdomen), with monitoring, may be considered. The 2019 Global Consensus Statement discourages compounded preparations except where no equivalent alternatives exist; efficacy and safety vary. *Adverse effects*: These include hirsutism and acne (generally mild), and rarely virilization (deepening of voice, clitoromegaly), usually linked to excessive dosing. *Contraindications*: These include cardiovascular or hepatic disease, endometrial or breast hyperplasia, or cancer. AT may involve estrogen-related risks (e.g., breast cancer, abnormal uterine bleeding); long-term safety is not established. Discontinue if no response is observed within 6 months. Injectable or implant formulations are contraindicated due to supraphysiological peaks and reversibility issues [20–23].

Nonhormonal pharmacological treatment

The rationale is based on the modulation of central neurotransmitters involved in sexual motivation and reward.

- **Flibanserin 100 mg PO at bedtime (Addyi®):** a 5-HT1A agonist and 5-HT2A antagonist, with partial dopaminergic agonist activity (D4). It increases norepinephrine/dopamine release and reduces serotonin in the cortex, restoring prefrontal control over motivation/reward circuits and facilitating desire arousal. Approved by the FDA for premenopausal women; not approved by ANVISA (unavailable in Brazil) [24].

- **Bremelanotide 1.75 mg SC on demand (~45 min before intercourse):** a melanocortin agonist indicated for premenopausal women. *Common adverse effects*: nausea/vomiting (limits acceptability). Not approved by ANVISA; unavailable in Brazil [25].

- **Bupropion 150 mg/day PO:** dopamine/norepinephrine reuptake inhibitor and 5-HT2 blocker, with mild-to-moderate prosexual effect. Useful in HSDD associated with antidepressants ("antidote" strategy). Contraindicated in epilepsy, bulimia, and anorexia [26].

- **Tribulus terrestris 280 mg PO daily** (equivalent to 112 mg of protodioscin) for 90–120 days: herbal medicine approved by ANVISA in Brazil. The phytocomplex (including protodioscin) mimics 5-α-reductase, favoring the conversion of testosterone into dihydrotestosterone (DHT); DHT may increase the LH peak and activate nitric oxide in nerve endings during genital arousal, promoting vaginal congestion. A safe and potentially effective option for women during reproductive years, perimenopause, and postmenopause [27, 28].

6.5 Nonpharmacological treatments

- **Sex therapy (ST):** It is a brief, specialized approach to relational obstacles (communication, routine, intimacy, cultural/religious beliefs). It includes education on the sexual response cycle, agreement on acceptable frequency when interests diverge, and sensate focus exercises: starting with nongenital touch (Focus 1), progressing to genital touch (Focus 2), and finally sexual intercourse, always advancing after success at each stage [29].

- **Cognitive-behavioral therapy (CBT):** It integrates ST techniques into a broader framework, aiming to restructure beliefs (e.g., unrealistic expectations), reduce avoidance behaviors, and redirect attention from performance/anxiety to pleasure/spontaneity (self-exploration; focusing on arousing erotic stimuli). Psycho-sexual education is central to redefining the understanding of desire and sexual activity [30].

7. Final considerations

HSDD represents one of the greatest contemporary challenges in women's sexual health, given its high prevalence, multidimensional impact, and persistent barriers to diagnosis and treatment. Recognizing it not merely as a clinical condition but as a biopsychosocial phenomenon is essential to reduce stigma and legitimize women's suffering.

Its pathophysiology shows that sexual desire results from a dynamic balance between excitatory and inhibitory systems, modulated by neurotransmitters, hormones, psychological factors, and relational dynamics. This integrative model reinforces the need for comprehensive diagnostic approaches capable of identifying everything from biological causes to cultural elements that limit erotic expression.

In management, the importance lies in the following:

- Validating the complaint as legitimate and relevant, countering feelings of guilt or inadequacy;

- Educating the patient and the couple, explaining the normalcy of spontaneous and responsive desire, and promoting erotic communication tools (attention, trust, and autonomy); and

- Adopting multimodal strategies, including safe, evidence-based pharmacological therapies alongside psychotherapeutic and relational interventions.

In sum, the treatment of HSDD should not be seen as a mere pharmacological prescription, but as an opportunity to reconstruct female sexuality in its entirety – biological, psychological, relational, and cultural. Clinical practice must be supported by scientific evidence, yet guided by sensitive listening, individualized interventions, and the recognition of sexuality as a fundamental dimension of health and quality of life.

Author details

Fabiene Bernardes Castro Vale[1,2*] and Laura de Siqueira Khouri[3]

1 Professor, Faculty of Medicine, Department of Gynecology and Obstetrics, Federal University of Minas Gerais (UFMG), Belo Horizonte, Brazil

2 PhD and MSc in Women's Health, Federal University of Minas Gerais (UFMG), Belo Horizonte, Brazil

3 Medical Student, Faculty of Medicine, Pontifical Catholic University of Minas Gerais (PUC Minas), Belo Horizonte, Brazil

*Address all correspondence to: fabienebcv@yahoo.com.br

References

[1] McCabe MP, Sharlip ID, Atalla E, Balon R, Fisher AD, Laumann E, et al. Definitions of sexual dysfunctions in women and men: A consensus statement from the Fourth international consultation on sexual medicine 2015. The Journal of Sexual Medicine. 2016;**13**:135–143

[2] Shifren JL, Monz BU, Russo PA, Segreti A, Johannes CB. Sexual problems and distress in United States women: Prevalence and correlates. Obstetrics & Gynecology. 2008;**112**(5):970–978

[3] West SL, D'Aloisio AA, Agans RP, Kalsbeek WD, Borisov NN, Thorp JM. Prevalence of low sexual desire and hypoactive sexual desire disorder in a nationally representative sample of US women. Archives of Internal Medicine. 2008;**168**(13):1441–1449

[4] Cacioppo S. Neuroimaging of female sexual desire and hypoactive sexual desire disorder. Sexual Medicine Reviews. 2017;**5**(4):434–444

[5] Pfaus JG. Pathways of sexual desire. The Journal of Sexual Medicine. 2009;**6**(6):1506–1533

[6] Calabro RS, Cacciola A, Bruschetta D, Milardi D, Quattrini F, Sciarrone F, et al. Neuroanatomy and function of human sexual behavior: A neglected or unknown issue? Brain and Behavior. 2019;**9**:e01389

[7] Salamone JD, Pardo M, Yohn SE, Lopez-Cruz L, SanMiguel N, Correa M. Mesolimbic dopamine and the regulation of motivated behavior. Current Topics in Behavioral Neurosciences. 2016;**27**:231–257

[8] Kruger THC, Keil L, Jung S, Kahl KG, Wittfoth M, Leeners B, et al. Lack of increase in sexual drive and function after dopaminergic stimulation in women. Journal of Sex & Marital Therapy. 2018;**44**:61–72

[9] Micevych PE, Meisel RL. Integrating neural circuits controlling female sexual behavior. Frontiers in Systems Neuroscience. 2017;**11**:42

[10] Inoue S. Hormonal and circuit mechanisms controlling female sexual behavior. Frontiers in Neural Circuits. 2024;**18**:1409349

[11] Gouveia M, Sanches R, Andrade S, Carmona S, Ferreira C. The role of testosterone in the improvement of sexual desire in postmenopausal women: An evidence-based clinical review. Acta Médica Portuguesa. 2018;**31**(11):680–690

[12] Ronghe R, Sengupta S, Chaudhari HK. Understanding hypoactive sexual desire disorder (HSDD) in women: Etiology, diagnosis, and treatment. Cureus. 2023;**15**(2): e35165. DOI: 10.7759/cureus.35165

[13] Seftel AD. Re: hypoactive sexual desire disorder: International Society for the Study of Women's Sexual Health (ISSWSH) expert consensus panel review. The Journal of Urology. 2017;**198**(2):235

[14] Clayton AH, Goldfischer ER, Goldstein I, Derogatis L, Lewis-D'Agostino DJ, Pyke R. Validation of the decreased sexual desire screener (DSDS): A brief diagnostic instrument for generalized acquired female hypoactive sexual desire disorder

(HSDD). The Journal of Sexual Medicine. 2009;**6**(3):730–738

[15] Clayton AH, Kingsberg SA, Goldstein I. Evaluation and management of hypoactive sexual desire disorder. Sexual Medicine. 2018;**6**(2):59–74

[16] Kingsberg SA, Althof S, Simon JA, Bradford A, Bitzer J, Carvalho J, et al. Female sexual dysfunction—medical and psychological treatments, Committee 14. The Journal of Sexual Medicine. 2017;**14**:1463–1491

[17] Lynn M, Mumby P. Response to letter to the editor: Reflections on "multidisciplinary approach to the treatment of sexual dysfunction in couples using a biopsychosocial model". The Journal of Sexual Medicine. 2023;**20**(10):1263

[18] Brotto LA, Atallah S, Carvalho J, Gordon E, Pascoal PM, Reda M, et al. Psychological and interpersonal dimensions of sexual function and dysfunction: Recommendations from the fifth international consultation on sexual medicine (ICSM 2024). Sexual Medicine Reviews. 2025;**13**:118–143

[19] Genazzani AR, Pluchino N, Bernardi F, Centofanti M, Luisi M. Beneficial effect of tibolone on mood, cognition, well-being, and sexuality in menopausal women. Neuropsychiatric Disease and Treatment. 2006;**2**(3): 299–307

[20] Worsley R, Santoro N, Miller KK, Parish SJ, Davis SR. Hormones and female sexual dysfunction: Beyond estrogens and androgens–findings from the fourth international consultation on sexual medicine. The Journal of Sexual Medicine. 2016;**13**(3):283–290

[21] Davis SR, Baber R, Panay N, Bitzer J, Cerdas Perez S, Islam RM, et al. Global consensus position statement on the use of testosterone therapy for women. Climacteric. 2019;**22**:429–434

[22] Jang C, Boyle JA, Vincent A. Global consensus statement on testosterone therapy for women: An Australian perspective. Medical Journal of Australia. 2020;**213**(10):449–52e1

[23] Parish SJ, Simon JA, Davis SR, Giraldi A, Goldstein I, Goldstein SW, et al. International society for the study of women's sexual health clinical practice guideline for the use of systemic testosterone for hypoactive sexual desire disorder in women. The Journal of Sexual Medicine. 2021;**18**:849–867

[24] Katz M, DeRogatis LR, Ackerman R, Hedges P, Lesko L, Garcia Jr M, et al. Begonia trial investigators. Efficacy of flibanserin in women with hypoactive sexual desire disorder: Results from the BEGONIA trial. The Journal of Sexual Medicine. 2013;**10**:1807–1815

[25] Kingsberg SA, Clayton AH, Portman D, Williams LA, Krop J, Jordan R, et al. Bremelanotide for the treatment of hypoactive sexual desire disorder: Two randomized phase 3 trials. Obstetrics & Gynecology. 2019;**134**:899–908

[26] Segraves RT, Clayton A, Croft H, Wolf A, Warnock J. Bupropion sustained-release for the treatment of hypoactive sexual desire disorder in premenopausal women. Journal of Clinical Psychopharmacology. 2004;**24**(3):339–342

[27] Stefanescu R, Tero-Vescan A, Negroiu A, Aurica E, Vari CE.

A comprehensive review of the phytochemical, pharmacological, and toxicological properties of Tribulus terrestris L. Biomolecules. 2020;**10**(5):752

[28] Ghanbari A, Akhshi N, Nedaei SE, Mollica A, Aneva IY, Qi Y, et al. Tribulus terrestris and female reproductive system health: A comprehensive review. Phytomedicine. 2021;**84**:153462

[29] Beasley CC, Ager R. Emotionally focused couples therapy: A systematic review of its effectiveness over the past 19 years. Journal of Evidence-Based Social Work. 2019;**16**(2):144–159

[30] Pyke RE, Clayton AH. Psychological treatment trials for hypoactive sexual desire disorder: A sexual medicine critique and perspective. The Journal of Sexual Medicine. 2015;**12**(12):2451–2458

Chapter 7

Sexual Dysfunction Among Women with Type 2 Diabetes Mellitus

Perianayagi Palavesam, Manopriya Thiruvagounder, Shankar Shanmugam Rajendran and Dhastagir Sultan Sheriff

Abstract

Female sexual dysfunction is prevalent among women with diabetes, further impacting their reproductive health and lifespan. Globally, female sexual dysfunction affects approximately 56.6% of women, with sexual desire disorder being the most prevalent (46.5%), followed by desire (interest) dysfunction (36.6%). Prolonged hyperglycemia increases the risk of infection, endothelial dysfunction, vascular damage, and neural damage, all of which contribute to sexual dysfunction. Hormonal imbalances and the psychological impact of living with diabetes, metformin, and lifestyle play crucial roles in sexual dysfunction. Metformin enhances uterine vascularity and blood flow by increasing insulin-like growth factor-binding protein-1 and glycodelin levels in the uterus. Healthcare providers should regularly discuss sexual health issues with women with diabetes, promote awareness, and address obstacles linked to female sexual dysfunction. Improved metabolic control often correlates with enhanced sexual function, and lifestyle modifications play a crucial role in effective diabetes management. Counseling therapy should be integrated into the management plan for women with diabetes experiencing sexual dysfunction.

Keywords: diabetes, female sexual dysfunction, organic causes, psychological, life style, metformin

1. Introduction

Sexual dysfunction is a significant complication of diabetes mellitus (DM) and can be an early indicator of the disease. In women, the causes of sexual dysfunction can be psychological or organic, with organic causes further categorized into gynecological and non-gynecological factors. Hormonal imbalances and autonomic neuropathies, which are common in DM, are frequent non-gynecological causes of sexual dysfunction (Samuel et al., 2022 [1]).

The global prevalence of DM has increased over the past decades, with estimates suggesting that it will affect 578 million adults by 2030 and 700 million by 2045. The estimated prevalence was similar in women and men aged 20–79 (10.9% vs. 11.3%).

According to the International Diabetes Federation (IDF) Diabetes Atlas, in 2021, approximately 9.8 million more men than women were diagnosed with diabetes.

The increasing prevalence of type 2 DM (T2DM) has been paralleled by a decrease in the average age of menarche. This association may be linked to lifestyle and environmental changes, as well as underlying biological processes. Sexual dysfunction affects a significant proportion of women with diabetes, further impacting their reproductive lifespan. Recognizing the correlation between reproductive health and T2DM is crucial.

Female sexual disorders/dysfunction (FSD) affect women across various reproductive stages, including the perimenopausal, menopausal, and postmenopausal stages. The interplay between biological and psychosocial factors influences human sexual response, with cultural, individual, and situational variations.

Despite evolving research, the prevalence of FSD remains relatively stable, affecting approximately 40%–50% of women. Women with T2DM are disproportionately affected, with a prevalence of 20%–80% compared to 40% in the general female population [2].

The global prevalence of FSD is approximately 56.6% (95% confidence interval [CI]: 47%–64%), with sexual desire disorder being the most common (46.5%), followed by desire (interest) dysfunction (36.6%) [3].

2. Factors contributing to FSD

Factors contributing to FSD in women with T2DM include:

- Longer diabetes duration (≥10 years): 2.87 times higher risk of poor sexual function;
- Poor glycemic control (higher glycated hemoglobin);
- Insulin therapy;
- Obesity (higher BMI);
- Advanced age;
- Earlier development of T2DM, influencing blood glucose management (Samuel et al., 2022 [1]).

These factors highlight the complex interplay between diabetes, metabolic control, and reproductive health in women with T2DM.

3. Classification of FSD

The American Psychiatric Association's DSM-5 (2013) categorizes FSD into three main categories (see **Table 1**).

S.No	Categories of FSD
1	Sexual interest/Arousal disorder
2	Orgasmic disorder
3	Genito-pelvic pain/Penetration disorder

Table 1.
Female sexual dysfunction categories as per the American Psychiatric Association's DSM-5 (2013).

(1) *Sexual interest/Arousal disorder:* Characterized by at least three symptoms, including reduced sexual interest, infrequent sexual thoughts or fantasies, lack of initiation of sexual activity, and reduced excitement or pleasure during sex. Symptoms must be present for at least six months and cause significant distress to the patient.

(2) *Orgasmic disorder:* Marked by delayed, infrequent, or absent orgasms, or reduced intensity of orgasms.

(3) *Genito-pelvic pain/Penetration disorder:* Characterized by difficulties with vaginal penetration, pain during intercourse, anxiety or fear related to penetration, or marked tightening of pelvic floor muscles [4].

The International Society for the Study of Women's Sexual Health has identified four key FSD categories (see **Table 2**).

(1) Hypoactive sexual desire disorder (HSDD) characterized by a decreased interest in sex and/or receptivity to a partner's initiation.

(2) Female sexual arousal disorder encompasses:

- Female cognitive arousal disorder (mental/emotional arousal difficulties)

- Female genital arousal disorder (genital arousal response issues)

(3) Persistent genital arousal disorder characterized by unwanted, intrusive genital arousal feelings.

(4) Female orgasm disorder characterized by compromised orgasm frequency or intensity.

S.No	Categories of FSD
1	Hypoactive sexual desire disorder (HSDD)
2	Female sexual arousal disorder
3	Persistent genital arousal disorder
4	Female orgasm disorder

Table 2.
Female sexual dysfunction categories as per the International Society for the Study of Women's Sexual Health.

4. Type 2 diabetes and reproductive function

4.1 Hypothalamic–pituitary–gonadal axis

T2DM is predominantly characterized by insulin resistance (IR) and hyperinsulinemia, which has already been mentioned to exacerbate gonadotropin-releasing hormone (GnRH) secretion, resulting in increased levels of luteinizing hormone (LH)/ follicle-stimulating hormone (FSH). These factors stimulate follicular development, induce ovarian stromal hyperplasia, and augment androgen biosynthesis. In addition to insulin, hormones secreted by adipose tissue have also been implicated. Hence, leptin stimulates GnRH production through kisspeptin, while adiponectin and ghrelin inhibit GnRH production. In contrast, Neuropeptide Y (NPY) stimulates or inhibits GnRH secretion depending on the patient's metabolic status (i.e., negative energy balance promotes the inhibition of GnRH secretion). Nevertheless, the exact role of these hormones in HPG function and the factors that regulate their circulating levels remain unclear [5].

4.2 Ovarian function

T2DM impairs normal ovarian function as IR and compensatory hyperinsulinemia stimulate excessive production of insulin-like growth factor-1 (IGF-1) and upregulate hybrid insulin/IGF-1 receptors. As a result, ovarian granulosa cells are stimulated, abnormal folliculogenesis is induced, and enlarged ovaries with multiple small follicles (characterized by polycystic ovarian morphology) develop. IGF receptor overactivity leads to higher production of ovarian androgens, as insulin maintains its action on the ovary, resulting in clinical hyperandrogenism in women with T2DM. Additionally, high insulin concentrations, acting as gonadotropins on theca cells of the ovaries, inhibit the recruitment of one dominant follicle, leading to menstrual disturbances and anovulation [6].

4.3 Development of polycystic ovarian syndrome in women with T2DM

Polycystic ovarian syndrome (PCOS) and T2DM appear to have a bidirectional relationship. PCOS is often characterized by IR and secretion defects, which contribute to glucose intolerance, particularly in obese individuals. Approximately 50% of women with PCOS exhibit IR linked to increased serine phosphorylation of the insulin receptor, which is mediated by a serine/threonine kinase. This mechanism affects insulin receptor signaling and androgen synthesis via P450c17 activity.

IR plays a significant role in the development of PCOS, affecting various tissues and hormonal pathways in the body. An inadequate response to insulin characterizes IR and can affect lean patients, not just those with adiposity. In women with PCOS, IR is tissue-specific, affecting skeletal muscles, adipocytes, and hepatocytes, while the ovaries and adrenal glands remain sensitive. Insulin stimulates androgen production in the ovaries, enhancing steroidogenesis and follicle growth. Hyperinsulinemia amplifies LH-binding sites, increases androgen response to LH, and reduces SHBG levels, leading to increased androgen production. Additionally, hyperinsulinemia inhibits IGF-1 binding protein synthesis, impairing granulosa cell survival and folliculogenesis. Chronic inflammation, marked by elevated white blood cell counts, CRP levels, and inflammatory biomarkers, contributes to the development of PCOS, with hyperandrogenism being a major contributor. Inflammatory cytokines such as tumor necrosis factor alpha (TNF-α) and interleukin 1 (IL-1) interfere with insulin signaling, suppress follicle development and ovulation, and exacerbate IR and PCOS symptoms. Overall, IR and hyperinsulinemia contribute to androgen excess, follicular dysfunction, and PCOS symptoms, while inflammation further impairs folliculogenesis and contributes to PCOS pathogenesis [7].

4.4 Fertility and T2DM

Women with T2DM have an increased risk of infertility. The risk of infertility increases with poor glycemic control and the presence of diabetic complications, as ovarian reserves deteriorate and antral follicle count declines [8].

4.5 Circadian clocks and fertility

The impact of modern lifestyle on fertility is significant, with stress disrupting the hypothalamic–pituitary–gonadal axis and affecting reproductive health. Clock genes regulate fertility in both men and women, and their disrupted expression can lead to decreased sex hormones, failed embryo implantation, and smaller newborn sizes.

The circadian clock controls metabolic variations that influence insulin release and glucose uptake. Even in the fasting state, insulin release follows a circadian rhythm. Disruptions, such as shift work, alter leptin, glucose, and insulin levels, contributing to metabolic issues. Metabolic signals, including insulin, also regulate circadian function, highlighting the complex interplay between metabolism and circadian rhythms [8].

5. T2DM and FSD

Prolonged hyperglycemia causes cellular damage via advanced glycation end-products (AGEs) and oxidative stress, affecting the vascular and brain tissues involved in sexual response. This leads to endothelial dysfunction, nerve damage, and decreased vaginal lubrication, all of which contribute to sexual dysfunction.

Hyperglycemia also increases the risk of infection, causes vaginal dryness, and exacerbates vascular and neural damage. Stable glycemic control is crucial for mitigating these effects.

Chronic inflammation, endothelial dysfunction, and cardiovascular disease are interconnected and contribute to sexual dysfunction in diabetes. Reduced nitric oxide bioavailability and impaired endothelial signaling decrease vaginal blood flow and lubrication.

Diabetes-related neuropathy affects sensory and autonomic neurons, reducing sensitivity and altering the genital reflexes. Atherosclerosis and cardiovascular diseases can also compromise genital blood flow, leading to similar sexual dysfunction symptoms.

Hormonal imbalances, particularly altered sex hormone levels, contribute to diminished sexual desire, vaginal dryness, and poor genital responsiveness in women.

The psychosocial impact of diabetes management can lead to anxiety, depression, and body image issues, exacerbating sexual dysfunction and straining relationships. A longer diabetes duration worsens these changes, emphasizing the need for early assessment and intervention [2].

6. Role of metformin in fertility

Metformin, a hydrophilic biguanide, is distributed in various tissues, including the hypothalamus, pituitary, and gonads, in addition to its well-known presence in the liver, pancreas, and adipose tissues. It can accumulate in specific tissues, such as the reproductive system, at higher concentrations than in the plasma through specific transport mechanisms.

Metformin activates AMP-activated protein kinase (AMPK), a key enzyme involved in cellular energy homeostasis. In the hypothalamus, AMPK influences the secretion of GnRH, which stimulates the pituitary gland to produce FSH and LH. As an AMPK activator, metformin decreases the amplitude of FSH and LH secretion through this pathway.

7. Metformin and FSD

Metformin plays a crucial role in PCOS pathogenesis amelioration, with extensive research supporting its efficacy. However, its application in non-PCOS infertile or sub-fertile women has not been extensively studied. IR, a common factor in conditions such as stress, aging, obesity, depression, and a sedentary lifestyle, can significantly affect fertility. Infertile women often present with one or more of these conditions, along with ovarian dysfunction, which can trigger a stress response mechanism, abnormal cortisol secretion, and increased catecholamine levels.

Metformin may offer benefits in these scenarios by enhancing uterine vascularity and blood flow through increased IGF-1 and increased glycodelin levels.

Metformin's potential mechanisms include:

- Enhancing FSH effectiveness via IGF-1-mediated granulosa cell growth regulation;

- Regulating steroidogenesis by reducing progesterone, estradiol, and androstenedione secretion from granulosa and theca cells [9].

8. Healthcare services and the role of healthcare professionals

Healthcare professionals should prioritize discussing sexual health in routine evaluations, as it is often neglected. This includes taking routine sexual anamnesis, incorporating sexual history in evaluations for women with type 2 diabetes, and addressing personal barriers such as taboos and confidentiality concerns. Providers should be trained to evaluate and address women's sexual function, adopting a multidisciplinary approach involving psychiatrists and sex therapists, if needed, for the comprehensive management of sexual dysfunction.

Managing FSD in women with diabetes involves a comprehensive approach that addresses the underlying diabetes-related factors and specific sexual concerns.

8.1 Optimizing glycemic control

Improved metabolic control is often correlated with better sexual functions. This can be achieved through diabetes management, including adherence to medication regimens, monitoring blood sugar levels, and making healthy lifestyle choices. Regular check-ups with healthcare providers are crucial for adjusting treatment plans as required.

8.2 Lifestyle modifications

Making healthy lifestyle changes can improve glycemic control and sexual health in patients with DM. Regular exercise boosts insulin sensitivity and enhances overall well-being. Quitting smoking reduces cardiovascular risk and improves blood flow. Stress reduction techniques, such as meditation, yoga, and therapy, can also help manage stress.

8.3 Specific treatments

Several treatments can address specific sexual problems. Vaginal moisturizers and lubricants help alleviate vaginal dryness and discomfort during sex. Pelvic floor physical therapy addresses dyspareunia and improves pelvic floor muscle function. Medications such as PDE-5 inhibitors (e.g., sildenafil and tadalafil) may improve blood flow and sexual responses. Other medications can address low libido or arousal problems.

8.4 Hormonal therapy

In postmenopausal women, hormone therapy may be considered after careful risk assessment. Estrogen therapy can improve vaginal lubrication and elasticity, whereas testosterone therapy may be considered for low libido.

8.5 PDE-5 inhibitors

These medications, commonly used for erectile dysfunction in men, have been studied in women with diabetes. They increase blood flow to the genital tissues, potentially improving the sexual response. Drugs like sildenafil, tadalafil, and vardenafil are examples. While studies suggest potential benefits, more research is needed to confirm their efficacy in women [10].

8.6 Improving care

Creating a secure environment and increasing healthcare provider awareness can help address women's sexual issues, ultimately benefiting their overall well-being [11].

Sexual dysfunction is a common issue among women with diabetes, and healthcare providers should address it in routine discussions. Factors such as depression, lack of physical activity, and complications or comorbidities are linked to sexual dysfunction and can be modified with appropriate care [3].

Holistic counseling therapy can improve sexual function and quality of life by addressing the physical, psychological, cultural, and individual aspects. Healthcare providers should consider incorporating counseling therapy into the care plan for women with diabetes who experience sexual dysfunction (Juliani et al., 2025 [12]).

9. Prevention and future management direction

Preventing FSD in women with diabetes involves maintaining optimal blood sugar control, early detection of complications, and addressing the modifiable risk factors (see **Figure 1**). Regular screening for sexual concerns should be part of routine diabetes care to enable early interventions.Prevention of sexual dysfunction.

The prognosis varies depending on factors such as age, duration and severity of diabetes, complications, and the effectiveness of interventions. Research shows that early intervention and comprehensive management can improve sexual function and quality of life among women with T2DM (see **Figure 2**).Sexual well-being among women with T2DM.

Emerging research areas include novel therapies, such as growth factors for vaginal health, new drug delivery systems, and psychological interventions.

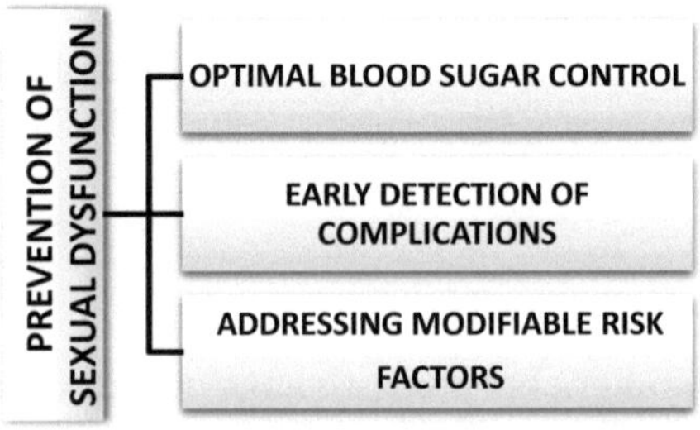

Figure 1.
Prevention of sexual dysfunction.

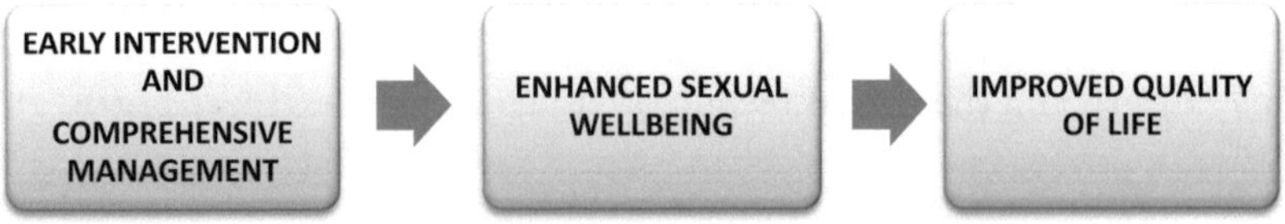

Figure 2.
Sexual well-being among women with T2DM.

Pharmacological options include ospemifene for vulvovaginal atrophy and flibanserin for HSDD. Future management may involve personalized medicine approaches based on individual risk factors and response patterns.

There is a growing need to integrate sexual healthcare into diabetes management programs and train healthcare providers to address these concerns. The development of new assessment tools and treatments for women with FSD is an active area of research. Understanding long-term intervention outcomes and predicting treatment success factors remain key research goals [10].

10. Conclusion

As DM becomes an increasingly significant burden with numerous complications, women with diabetes in the reproductive age group are not exempt from its effects on fertility. Sexual dysfunction in women with diabetes is less understood and addressed than it is in men. Educating healthcare professionals and training them to regularly assess and manage sexual dysfunction alongside disease management are crucial for improving the quality of life of women with diabetes.

Author details

Perianayagi Palavesam[1], Manopriya Thiruvagounder[2], Shankar Shanmugam Rajendran[3] and Dhastagir Sultan Sheriff[4]*

1 Department of Community Health Nursing, College of Nursing, Madras Medical College, Chennai, India

2 Dhanalakshmi Srinivasan Medical College and Hospital, Samayapuram, Tiruchi, India

3 College of Nursing, Madras Medical College, Chennai, India

4 Anna Medical College, Mauritius

*Address all correspondence to: drdsheriff@gmail.com

References

[1] Samuel et al. Sexual dysfunction among women with Diabetes Mellitus in a Nigerian Tertiary Hospital. International Journal of scientific research and review 2022;**5**:2998-3004

[2] Rogoznica M, Perica D, Borovac B, Belančić A, Matovinović M. Sexual Dysfunction in Female Patients with Type 2 Diabetes Mellitus—Sneak Peek on an Important Quality of Life Determinant. Diabetology. 2023;**4**(4):527–536. DOI: 10.3390/diabetology4040046

[3] Asefa A, Nigussie T, Henok A, Mamo Y. Prevalence of sexual dysfunction and related factors among diabetes mellitus patients in Southwest Ethiopia. BMC Endocrine Disorders. 2019;**19**(1):141. DOI: 10.1186/s12902-019-0473-1

[4] Kaundal A, Renjhen P. Female sexual dysfunction: A review. International Journal of Reproduction, Contraception, Obstetrics and Gynecology. 2024;**13**(5):1351–1359. DOI: 10.18203/2320-1770.ijrcog20241098

[5] Zaimi M, Michalopoulou O, Stefanaki K, Kazakou P, Vasileiou V, Psaltopoulou T, Karagiannakis DS, Paschou SA. Gonadal dysfunction in women with diabetes mellitus. Endocrine. 2024;**85**(2):461–472. DOI: 10.1007/s12020-024-03729-z

[6] Thong EP, Codner E, Laven JSE, Teede H. Diabetes: A metabolic and reproductive disorder in women. The Lancet Diabetes & Endocrinology. 2020;**8**(2):134–149. DOI: 10.1016/S2213-8587(19)30345-6

[7] Hajam YA, Rather HA, Neelam KR, Basheer M, Reshi MS. A review on critical appraisal and pathogenesis of polycystic ovarian syndrome. Endocrine and Metabolic Science. 2024;**14**:100162. DOI: 10.1016/j.endmts.2024.100162

[8] Sarankhuu B-E, Gantsolmon E, Enkhtugs K, Sankhuu Y, Purevdorj C, Yu S-L, Park S-R, Byambasukh O, Kang J. Diabetes and Adverse Reproductive Outcomes in a Group of Mongolian Women: A Comparative Study with Non-Diabetic Subjects. Journal of Clinical Medicine. 2025;**14**(17):6344. DOI: 10.3390/jcm14176344

[9] Pourmatroud E. Metformin in Health Issues and Reproductive System. In: Metformin. London: IntechOpen; 2019. p. 167–169. DOI: 10.5772/intechopen.90465

[10] Navriya SC, Jain M, Yadav O, Chowdary RC. Sexual Dysfunction in Female Patients with Diabetes. In: Feingold KR, Ahmed SF, Anawalt B, Blackman MR, Boyce A, Chrousos G, Corpas E, de Herder WW, Dhatariya K, Dungan K, Hofland J, Kalra S, Kaltsas G, Kapoor N, Koch C, Kopp P, Korbonits M, Kovacs CS, Kuohung W, Wilson DP, editors. Endotext. MDText.com, Inc; 2000. Available from: https://www.ncbi.nlm.nih.gov/books/NBK612823/

[11] Elyasi F, Kashi Z, Tasfieh B, Bahar A, Khademloo M. Sexual Dysfunction in Women with Type 2 Diabetes Mellitus. Iranian Journal of Medical Sciences. 2015;**40**(3):206–213. Available from: https://pmc.ncbi.nlm.nih.gov/articles/PMC4430881/

[12] Navriya SC, Jain M, Yadav O, et al. Sexual Dysfunction in Female Patients

with Diabetes. [Updated 2025 Mar 7]. In: Feingold KR, Adler RA, Ahmed SF, et al., editors. Endotext [Internet]. South Dartmouth (MA): MDText.com, Inc; 2000. Updated 2025 Mar 7: https://www.ncbi.nlm.nih.gov/books/NBK612823/

Chapter 8

Lichen Sclerosus and Its Impact on Female Sexual Dysfunction: A Comprehensive Review

Ramona Ramasamy and Karishma Hemmady

Abstract

Lichen sclerosus is a chronic inflammatory dermatosis that predominantly occurs in postmenopausal women. Although any area of the skin can be affected, the primary areas involved are the clitoris, labia majora, labia minora, and the anogenital region, leading to genital architectural changes. The precise aetiology remains unclear; however, there is evidence to suggest a multifactorial origin involving genetic predisposition, autoimmunity, hormonal influences, microbiome alteration, trauma, and environmental factors. The physical changes can lead to pain, pruritus, and dyspareunia, contributing to reduced sexual function and heightened anxiety, ultimately decreasing the quality of life due to the impact on the patient's psychosocial health and interpersonal relationships. Prompt diagnosis and early initiation of high-dose topical corticosteroids can alleviate some of the impact on quality of life. Other treatment modalities, such as immunomodulatory treatments, surgical interventions, and adjunctive psychological and physical therapies, can be explored for a patient-centred approach. A multifaceted approach to treatment involving gynaecology, dermatology, and psychiatry is needed to address the physical and psychological impact of the disease. Lichen sclerosus follows a chronic relapsing course with potential for malignant transformation, necessitating lifelong follow-up. This chapter, presented as a literature review, aims to explore the pathophysiology, diagnostic strategies, therapeutic interventions, and its impact on female sexual and psychological health using an evidence-based approach to comprehensive management.

Keywords: dyspareunia, lichen sclerosus, anogenital health, vulvar dermatoses, genital dermatology, sexual dysfunction, sexual response

1. Introduction

Discovered in 1886 by Hallopeau and referred to by various names, 'lichen sclerosus' was coined as a term by the International Society for the Study of Vulvovaginal Disease in 1976 to replace various other terms such as kraurosis vulvae, guttate scleroderma, balanitis xerotica obliterans, white spot disease, and lichen sclerosus et atrophicus [1]. Lichen sclerosus (LS) is a chronic, progressive, inflammatory dermatological condition that predominantly affects women more than men. The ratios vary between 3:1 and 10:1 [2], with the mean age of onset being the fifth and sixth decades of life, and the youngest reported case being two years old [3]. It predominantly affects the anogenital region; however, there are a small number of cases where extragenital manifestations have been reported, most commonly on the breast and back [4]. The exact aetiology of LS has not been pinpointed; it is multifactorial, with hormonal status, frequent trauma, and autoimmune diseases as well-known associations for LS [5]. Whilst the wart virus and other infective pathologies have been suggested, no correlation has been found to support this evidence [3, 5]. LS can cause significant morbidity due to pruritus, pain, and anatomical disfigurement. Vulvar pain, which is one of the most reported symptoms by affected women, leads to sexual dysfunction and adversely affects their psyche, adding undue stress [6]. Due to the high prevalence of LS in postmenopausal women, LS represents an important area of study, underscoring the need to provide a holistic, patient-centred approach to treatment.

2. Pathophysiology and aetiology of lichen sclerosus

2.1 Overview of pathogenesis

The aetiology of LS remains unknown, but studies have suggested that it is polygenic in nature. Studies have identified genetic, autoimmune, hormonal, trauma, lifestyle choices, and infectious components as possible aetiologies. See **Table 1** below for the various aetiologies of lichen sclerosus.

2.2 Age and sex predisposition (males, children, females)

LS typically affects both males and females across all age groups, but females are generally more susceptible than males. The disease presents in two peak age groups for vulvar LS: prepubertal and postmenopausal years. Similarly, LS in males also shows a bimodal onset pattern, affecting young boys and adult men, which will not be further explored here [7].

2.3 Genetic factors

The genetic component of LS has been strongly associated with genes regulating HLA class II antigens, which influence hormonal activity. In particular, HLA-DQ7

Factor	Evidence/mechanism
Genetics	HLA associations (eg, HLA-DQ7); familial clustering.
Autoimmune mechanisms	Association with thyroiditis, vitiligo, alopecia; ECM1 antibodies.
Hormonal influences	Oestrogen deficiency, androgen receptor dysfunction.
Microbiome dysfunction	Altered vulvar flora, impaired barrier function.
Trauma	Koebner phenomenon, chronic irritation.
Environmental factors	Stress, infections, possible smoking, and obesity.

Table 1.
Multifactorial aetiology of lichen sclerosus.

has shown a high prevalence in individuals with LS. Evidence suggests that 50% of adult females, 45% of adult males, and 66% of prepubertal females with HLA-DQ7 have been diagnosed with LS [8]. Familial clustering has been demonstrated by studies, with approximately 10% of patients with lichen sclerosus having relatives with the same disease [9]. Whilst the mode of inheritance remains unknown, LS inheritance has been observed in monozygotic and dizygotic twins, siblings, and mother–daughter pairs [8].

2.4 Autoimmune mechanisms

Some experts believe LS to be an autoimmune disease. Circulating antibodies targeting extracellular matrix protein 1 (ECM1) and the basement membrane zone (mainly BP180 and BP230) have been found in LS. To further support the theory, LS is frequently prevalent with other autoimmune conditions [10].

One of the more commonly associated autoimmune conditions linked to LS is thyroid disorders. Whilst the exact pathological mechanisms behind the association remain unknown, both conditions are known to involve the abnormal activity of T lymphocytes. In patients with LS, autoreactive T cells against basement membrane proteins have been detected in both vulvar tissue and their peripheral blood samples. A similar type of immunological pattern is also noted in autoimmune thyroid disorders [11].

In vitiligo, it is suggested that inflammatory changes trigger an autoimmune reaction to melanocytes as the common immunogenic connection underlying the documented association of LS with vitiligo [12].

Research indicates that dysfunction of ECM1, found at the dermal–epidermal junction, has possible implications for the pathogenesis of LS. ECM1 is thought to act as the biological glue responsible for the structural organization and integrity of human skin. Therefore, when there is disruption to this layer by ECM1 autoantibodies, it results in pathologies such as LS. Evidence also suggests that ECM1 dysfunction in other skin pathologies, such as lipoid proteinosis, causes symptoms similar to LS [13].

2.5 Hormonal influences

Since lichen sclerosus (LS) largely follows a bimodal peak, its prevalence pattern affects women in their prepubertal and postmenopausal years. These peaks suggest that hypoestrogenism plays a key role in the development of LS [14]. A study by Eduard et al. suggests decreased levels of 5-α reductase (an enzyme that converts testosterone to dihydrotestosterone) as a possible cause. Patients with untreated LS had significantly higher levels of free testosterone and considerably lower levels of dihydrotestosterone and androstenedione in their serum when compared to normal levels for their age [15].

2.6 Microbiome and barrier dysfunction

Evidence shows that microbiome and barrier dysfunction can affect gynaecological health. Vaginal microbiome imbalance can cause chronic irritation, including increased inflammation and epithelial barrier damage; this, in turn, can lead to LS. A healthy vaginal microbiota typically contains a large number of Lactobacillus species. Studies have shown that a high number of non-Lactobacillus-dominant vulvar and vaginal microbiomes are observed in women with LS. A study by Taylor et al. showed that the vaginal and vulvar microbiomes in postmenopausal women with LS contained a high number of Actinomyces and Ezakiella, suggesting that these bacteria may play a role in the pathogenesis of LS [16].

2.7 Trauma

LS has been associated with trauma and irritation to the genital area, particularly related to surgery, sexual intercourse, tissue damage during childbirth, and genital jewellery and piercing [17]. The Koebner phenomenon (lesions of a preexisting dermatosis on areas of cutaneous injury) is observed in LS, as the condition has been seen to occur in areas with various injuries [18].

2.8 Environmental and lifestyle factors

When examining risk factors associated with LS, lifestyle factors should be considered. Whilst there is no conclusive evidence suggesting that stress is related to LS, patients with LS are often under stress from the challenge of navigating and coping with a chronic disease.

Studies have explored LS's association with lifestyle choices such as obesity, smoking, and even the level of education. An Italian study showed that individuals affected by LS were more likely to be overweight or obese when compared to the general Italian population. The study theorized that a higher level of education was linked to a sedentary lifestyle and lower physical activity, which, combined with metabolic factors, may predispose individuals to LS development [19].

Various studies have demonstrated increased cardiovascular risk factors amongst LS patients. These include type 2 diabetes mellitus and hypertension. The association between LS and cardiovascular risk factors is thought to be similar to that of other chronic inflammatory skin diseases. The inflammation and autoimmune nature of LS could increase the risk of diabetes mellitus. Pathogenesis likely involves changes in inflammatory molecules, such as cytokines and adipocytokines, which may contribute to diabetes in people with LS. Similarly, the microvascular damage caused by LS may lead to hypertension. Uncontrolled diabetes mellitus and hypertension can cause further microvascular injury, which in turn increases cardiovascular risk [20].

2.9 Summary of multifactorial aetiology

Whilst the aetiology of LS still remains unclear, it is fair to assume that it is multifactorial in nature. The pathogenesis involves a combination of genetic, autoimmune, hormonal, environmental, and infectious components. The common mechanisms in these components involve inflammation, tissue remodelling, and scarring, which are all hallmark characteristics of LS.

3. Clinical presentation and diagnosis

3.1 Typical symptoms/vulvar manifestations

Lichen sclerosus most commonly affects the anogenital region in women, causing substantial discomfort and changes to the vulvar architecture [6]. The primary symptom of vulvar LS is pruritus, an intense and persistent itching that is severe enough to cause sleep disturbances in the patient.

Other than the pruritus, patients can also experience pain, sexual dysfunction, and urinary and bowel symptoms. Erosions and fissures can occur due to lichen sclerosus (LS), which can lead to pain, soreness, and dysuria. This, in turn, leads to dyspareunia and apareunia. The architectural changes resulting from chronic inflammation can also cause vulval scarring. One of the main architectural changes that occur is the narrowing of the introitus, resulting in painful intercourse. The amalgamation of these symptoms consequently leads to sexual dysfunction [6, 21, 22]. When the perianal region is affected, anal fissures can develop due to chronic inflammation, and the pain during defecation can lead to constipation (32.5% according to one study) and bowel disorders [3, 21]. Urinary symptoms occur more commonly in males than in females; however, females more commonly report overactive bladder (15.3%) and stress urinary incontinence (27.9%) [21]. In women, LS often involves the vulva and the perianal skin, creating a characteristic 'figure-of-eight' or hourglass shape. The most affected sites include the interlabial sulci, labia minora, clitoral hood, and perineum [17, 21].

Vulvar manifestations

Vulvar LS typically starts around the periclitoral hood, usually with a sharply demarcated nonspecific erythema and prominent oedema. This progresses to the labia minora, vestibule, perineal, and perianal regions.

- **Primary lesions**: The condition typically begins with the appearance of flat, ivory, or porcelain-white spots or polygonal papules. Historically, this gave LS the name 'white-spot-disease' [22].

- **Plaques and patches**: These initial spots often merge to form larger patches or plaques that can appear thin, crinkled, or like cellophane [22].

- **Colour variation**: Whilst pallor is the most common sign, the skin can also exhibit areas of redness (erythema), hyperpigmentation, and bruising (ecchymoses or purpura). Telangiectasias (small, dilated blood vessels) may also be visible [21, 22].

- **Sequelae**: Clitoral phimosis can lead to the formation of painful smegmatic pseudocysts and adhesions [3].

Architectural changes and scarring

LS is a scarring condition that can cause profound and irreversible changes to the vulvar anatomy [3, 17].

- Loss of structures: The labia minora (inner lips) may shrink, flatten, and eventually become completely resorbed or fused [3, 17].

- Clitoral changes: Scar tissue can fuse the clitoral hood, 'burying' the clitoris and making it difficult or impossible to see. Adhesions of the clitoral hood can also lead to the formation of smegmatic pseudocysts [17, 21].

- Narrowing of the vaginal opening: Progressive scarring can lead to stenosis (narrowing) of the vaginal introitus, which contributes to sexual dysfunction [17, 21].

3.2 Clinical signs

Anogenital lichen sclerosus in females

Anogenital lichen sclerosus (LS) in females most commonly affects the interlabial sulci, labia minora, clitoral hood, perineum, and perianal skin. This distribution is referred to as the 'figure-of-eight' pattern around the vulva and anus [3].

Primary lesions and colour changes

- The disease may start with slightly elevated erythema (redness), particularly around the clitoral hood, and oedema (swelling) [17, 21].
- The primary lesions are typically flat, ivory-white or porcelain-white polygonal papules and macules. They may merge into larger patches or plaques [17, 22].
- Pallor (pale, whitish skin) and sclerosis (tight, yellowish-white, scarred skin) can be observed in the affected areas [21].
- The skin can become thin, atrophic, and crinkled, described as having a 'parchment-like' or 'cellophane paper' appearance [17, 21, 22].
- The chronic scratching and inflammation can also lead to hyperkeratosis or lichen simplex chronicus superimposed on LS, causing thickened, leathery skin [21, 22].
- Fragility of the skin is a hallmark sign, leading to purpura (purple spots) and ecchymoses (bruising), which are common and harmless but can be distressing [17, 21].
- The affected skin is fragile and prone to splitting, tearing, or forming open sores (erosions and ulcerations), especially at the posterior fourchette (the area between the vagina and anus), leading to fissures [17, 21].
- Whilst very rare, blistering can occur in the affected areas [21].

3.3 Extragenital manifestations

Whilst the most common area of manifestation of LS is the anogenital region, approximately 6–20% of patients show a predilection for extragenital regions, with females being affected more than males at a ratio of 6:1 to 10:1 [3, 10, 21, 23]. It is rarer still for LS to manifest solely as extragenital, and this has only been reported in 6% of cases [17, 23].

The extragenital variation has its own sequelae. Whilst starting similar to the anogenital variation with papules transforming into plaques, the next stage is follicular plugging. Follicular plugging refers to keratin clots that form within the hair follicles and resemble closed comedones [9, 17, 21]. The morphological variants include atrophic plaques, guttate lesions (small, discrete, raindrop-like hypopigmented macules), scleroatrophic lesions (shiny, porcelain-white atrophic plaques), and hyperkeratotic lesions (whitish, thickened plaques, some resembling comedones) [3, 24]. Rarer variants include bullous, ulcerative, annular, desquamative, telangiectatic, angiokeratomatous, verrucous, and vitiligoid forms [21]. See **table 2** for a more detailed overview of the clinical manifestations of extragenital lesions in LS.

Extragenital LS can appear on almost any part of the body, but certain areas are more commonly affected. The trunk (38.5%) is the most frequent site, followed by the lower extremities (23.1%), upper extremities (34.2%), and face (3.8%) [24]. The submammary area (under the breasts), neck, shoulders, upper back, chest, inner thighs, buttocks, wrists, and axillae are more commonly featured in the literature, whilst the head and scalp are rarer [3, 17, 21, 23, 24].

A key difference from genital LS is that extragenital lesions are usually asymptomatic; they rarely cause the pruritus or pain characteristic of anogenital LS. The lack of symptoms is thought to be due to the absence of occlusion, moisture, and friction that exacerbate the condition in the genital region. If symptoms do occur, they are typically mild pruritus [3, 9, 23, 24].

There is a strong association with the Koebner phenomenon; lesions have been observed to arise in places of scars from surgery, burns, or skin grafts, as well as sites of injury, tattooed skin, and areas of constant friction or pressure [9, 18, 21]. In rarer cases, they have been observed in Blaschko's lines, a linear band-like pattern that follows the invisible lines of skin development [21].

3.4 Paediatric presentations

LS has a bimodal age distribution, with peaks in prepubertal girls and postmenopausal women, with prepubertal girls making up 7–15% of VLS cases [25–28]. Whilst the underlying disease is the same, its presentation, long-term risks, and management differ significantly between these two groups. See **table 3** below for a detailed comparision between paediatric and adult LS.

System/region	Clinical manifestations
Skin (nongenital)	Porcelain-white atrophic plaques (commonly found on the trunk, neck, shoulders, upper arms, breasts, and thighs) see **Figure 1.** Hypopigmented patches with a wrinkled 'cigarette-paper' texture. Follicular plugging may be visible.
Oral mucosa	White, sclerotic plaques on the buccal mucosa, tongue, gingiva, and lips. Symptoms: burning, discomfort, restricted mobility (eg, tongue).
Oesophagus	Dysphagia due to strictures (rare).
Anus/perianal (outside classic vulvar/perianal LS)	White, sclerotic plaques perianally without genital involvement. Fissures, pain, and bleeding.
Scalp	White patches with follicular plugging. Potential scarring alopecia (rare).
Nails	Longitudinal ridging, thinning, and dystrophy.
Palms & soles	Hypopigmented or sclerotic plaques. Painful fissures are possible.
Breasts	Sclerotic, ivory-white plaques on the areola and breast tissue.

Table 2.
Extragenital manifestations.

Feature	Paediatric LS	Adult LS
Scarring	Less common than in adults (20% of girls), but it can occur with delayed diagnosis [26].	Very common and often severe, leading to anatomical changes and functional impairment (approximately 79% of women) [28].
Malignancy risk	No evidence of squamous cell carcinoma (SCC) developing in prepubertal lesions has been found. However, childhood-onset lichen sclerosus (LS) is a risk factor for developing SCC in adulthood [21, 25].	There is a 4–5% lifetime risk of developing vulvar or penile SCC on lesions [3].
Remission	Spontaneous remission may occur at puberty in about 25% of girls [27]. In boys, circumcision is often curative [9].	Remission is rare. Lifelong monitoring and maintenance therapy are required to control symptoms and prevent progression [3,9].

Table 3.
The long-term outlook for LS differs between paediatric and adult patients.

The most frequent symptoms are pruritus and soreness in the genital area in both adult and paediatric populations. However, children are more likely than adults to experience dysuria and pain during defecation, which can lead to secondary constipation as they withhold stool to avoid pain [3, 27]. The lesions appear as white, pearly, sclerotic plaques, often in a characteristic '**figure of eight"**' pattern around the vulva and anus. Purpura (bruising) is a hallmark feature in children and, combined with fissures, can be mistaken for sexual abuse, necessitating careful evaluation [25–27]. The white lesions, along with itching, burning, discomfort, vaginal bleeding, and dysuria, can potentially lead to misdiagnosis as sexually transmitted diseases in sexually active underage girls and potential abuse [26]. This can result in delays in diagnosis (between 1 and 1.6 years on average) and treatment, leading to more painful symptoms for the child [28].

LS is a primary cause of acquired phimosis in prepubertal boys and will not be explored in this chapter [27].

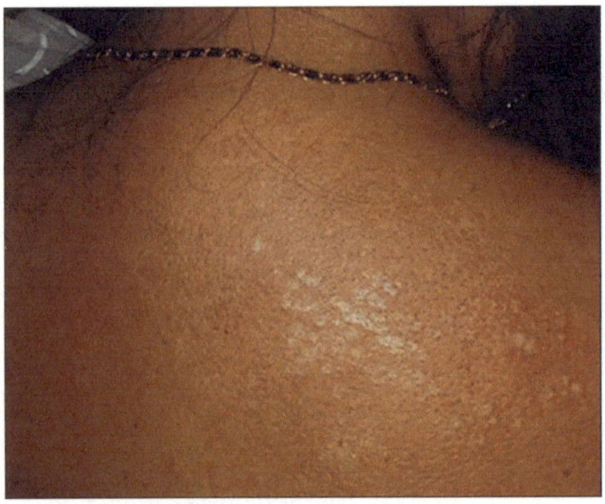

Figure 1.
Extragenital lichen sclerosus et atrophicus: grouped white macules on the back. Clinical photograph showing hypopigmented, plaques with a shiny surface over the upper back and shoulder region. The lesions exhibit areas of coalescence and irregular borders against surrounding normal skin.

3.5 Complications

If LS is left untreated or poorly managed, it can lead to significant and often debilitating complications. These complications can range from physical and anatomical changes, functional impairments, severe impacts on quality of life, and, most insidiously, malignant transformation to SCC.

Unlike anogenital LS, which carries a lifetime risk of 4–5% for developing SCC, extragenital LS is not associated with malignant transformation [3, 9, 18]. The transformation is thought to be driven by chronic inflammation, oxidative DNA damage, and alterations in tumour suppressor genes such as p53 [26]. SCC cases associated with LS have not been found to be positive for the oncogenic HPV virus [9]. Case studies of excised vulvar SCCs have found evidence of LS in the adjacent skin in up to 61% of cases [3]. There have been reports of superimposed lichen simplex due to chronic scratching, leading to subepithelial haemorrhage [17].

3.6 Differential diagnosis

It is critical to differentiate LS from other pathologies, as its symptoms and appearance, especially in early or atypical stages, can mimic a wide range of other disorders (See **Table 4**). The diagnosis is often clinical but may require a biopsy for definitive confirmation.

3.7 Diagnostic criteria and guidelines

The approach to diagnosis and long-term management is tailored to the patient's age. The most common method for diagnosing LS is through history, clinical symptoms, and physical examination. Guidelines recommend a high vaginal swab to rule out any sexually transmitted diseases and routine blood investigations,

Differential diagnosis	Clinical features
Lichen planus	Erosions of the vaginal introitus; reticulated white lines (Wickham's striae) at lesion edges [17] see **Figure 2.**
Vitiligo	Clearly defined depigmentation with no scarring and no symptoms [21].
Eczema	Erythema with scaling; lichenification (thickened skin) but no atrophic changes observed in LS [21].
Psoriasis	Erythema with well-demarcated silver scaling [26].
Morphea (localized scleroderma)	Involves deeper dermal and subcutaneous tissue, whilst LS is usually confined to the superficial (papillary) dermis [3].
Autoimmune blistering dermatosis	Erosions or blisters, which are rare in LS [17].
Malignancy	Lesions are often indurated and grow progressively [26].
Candida infection	Redness and characteristic white, atrophic changes of LS are absent [21].
Trauma or sexual abuse (children)	Extragenital findings are present [3].

Table 4.
Differential diagnosis of vulvar lichen sclerosus.

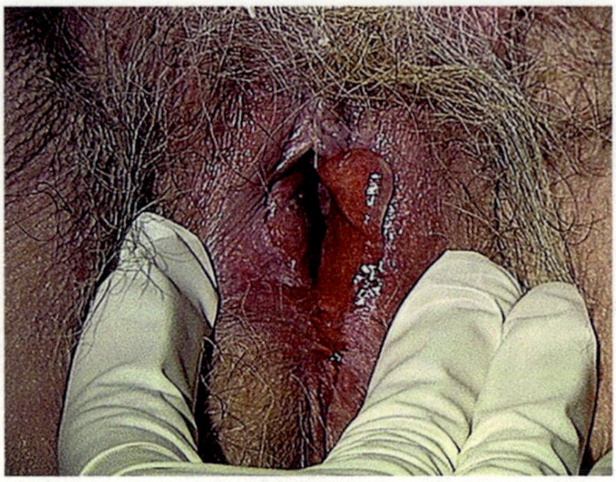

(a)

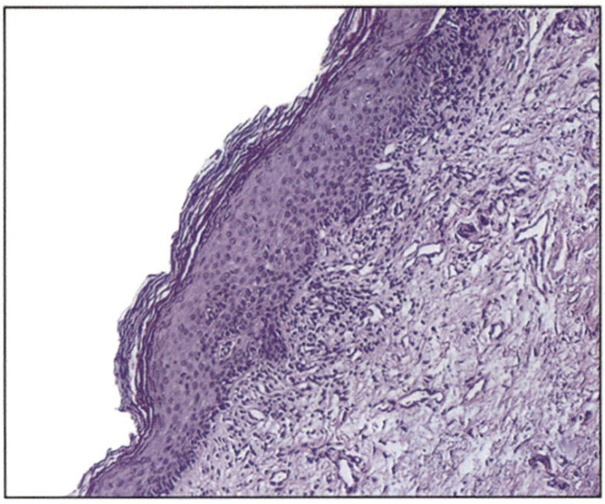

(b)

Figure 2.
Wide vestibular erythematous erosive lichen planus in a 79-year-old woman. (b) Representative example of a lichen planus biopsy specimen showing irregular hyperkeratosis and a lymphoid dermal infiltrate appearing as a distinct band close to the epidermis. Affiliation: Department of Gynecology and Obstetrics, Regional Hospital Citadelle, 4000 Liège, Belgium. Source: Open Access MedlinePlus.

including HbA1c for pruritus [29]. Biopsy is often performed in adults to confirm the diagnosis, rule out malignancy, and establish a baseline for monitoring [21, 25, 27]. In children, the diagnosis is primarily clinical, and biopsy is avoided due to the traumatic nature of the procedure in the genital area and the absence of cancer risk [21, 25, 27].

3.8 Histopathology

The classic presentation of LS is characterized by a 'red, white, and blue' pattern on low-power magnification, which corresponds to three key changes in the skin layers: hyperkeratosis (red), dermal sclerosis (white), and a lymphocytic infiltrate (blue) [27].

These classic features can be broken down by skin layer (see **table 5**)

The histological presentation of LS changes as the disease progresses.

Skin layer	Histopathologic manifestations
Epidermis (top layer)	Hyperkeratosis: thickening of the outermost layer of the stratum corneum. Epidermal atrophy: thinning of the living layers of the epidermis. Flattening of rete ridges: the loss of the normal wavelike projections of the epidermis into the dermis.
Dermoepidermal junction	Basal layer degeneration: damage to the deepest layer of the epidermis, often described as hydropic or vacuolar degeneration. Thickened basement membrane: though this can sometimes be difficult to distinguish from a thin layer of sclerosis.
Papillary dermis (upper dermis)	Sclerosis/hyalinization: a hallmark feature, which shows a pale-staining, 'ground glass' zone of homogenized, swollen collagen fibres. This zone is also associated with a loss of elastic fibres. Oedema: the sclerotic zone is often oedematous. Dilated vessels: frequently observed within or below the sclerotic band.
Reticular dermis (mid-dermis)	Band-like lymphocytic infiltrate: seen below the sclerotic zone, there is typically a dense, band-like infiltrate of inflammatory cells, mainly lymphocytes and some histiocytes.
Adnexal structures	Follicular plugging: Keratin plugs can be seen obstructing hair follicles, a common feature in nonmucosal skin and extragenital lichen sclerosus (LS).

Table 5.
Histopathological changes [3, 21, 27, 28].

Early presentation – presclerotic

The initial presentation is inflammatory and often lichenoid in nature, displaying a dense lymphocytic infiltrate at the dermal–epidermal junction. There may be mild and irregular psoriasiform thickening of the epidermis, but not atrophy. The histopathology can be difficult to distinguish from differentials such as lichen planus, psoriasis, or nonspecific dermatitis (eg, eczema). It is hard to make a firm diagnosis, such as LS, without clinical correlation, hence the term 'presclerotic' [17, 21, 27].

Sclerotic presentation – conventional

This is the classic presentation of LS, characterized by epidermal atrophy, a band of hyalinized, sclerotic collagen in the papillary dermis, and an inflammatory infiltrate that has been pushed further down and deeper below this area. The epidermis is flat and thin, although there may be pseudoepithelial hyperplasia in one or more areas [17, 21, 27].

Atrophic presentation – late

In late or 'burnt-out' lesions, the inflammatory infiltrate is often scant or absent, and prominent sclerosis is usually replaced by a less dense matrix of fibrosis, with the epidermis being extremely thin and atrophic [17, 21, 27].

Nonsclerotic lichen sclerosus (NSLS)

Many patients with true lichen sclerosus (LS), potentially one-third of all cases, may not exhibit dermal sclerosis in a biopsy specimen and are instead classified as having NSLS [30]. In these cases, the diagnosis of LS requires very strong clinical correlation; the pathology report will typically be descriptive and will not provide a definitive diagnosis.

NSLS could be separated into four major histopathological patterns:

1. Lichenoid dermatitis: This is the most common NSLS pattern, characterized by a band-like lymphocytic infiltrate and basal degeneration, but it does not exhibit sclerosis. The epidermis may range from atrophic to slightly thickened [30].

2. Hypertrophic lichenoid dermatitis: This condition is characterized by an acanthotic (thickened) epidermis, usually accompanied by hyperkeratosis and basal degeneration. It may be difficult to distinguish it from hypertrophic lichen planus or psoriasis [30].

3. Dermal fibrosis without acanthosis: This is the least common type, usually characterized by a normal or atrophic epidermis and dermal fibrosis rather than dermal sclerosis. It typically has a sparse inflammatory infiltrate and can be mistaken for a scar [30].

4. Dermal fibrosis with acanthosis: This pattern features a thickened, hyperkeratotic epidermis originating from the dermal fibrosis. A unique aspect is the presence of collagen bundles arranged horizontally, with intervening rows of lymphocytes emerging in a single file. The primary diagnosis would be lichen simplex chronicus [30].

3.9 Imaging and other tests

The diagnosis of lichen sclerosus is primarily clinical since the disease is a mucocutaneous disorder; its diagnosis is made through direct visualization and predominantly histopathology. Radiology does not play a role in the diagnosis of lichen sclerosus. Various tests are used in conjunction with history and examination to rule out other differentials rather than to confirm lichen sclerosus. The gold standard for diagnosing lichen sclerosus is histopathology; however, there are cases where it is avoided, such as in children with genital lesions, to prevent causing additional trauma [9].

Noninvasive diagnostic tools

These tools aid in clinical diagnosis and can sometimes reduce the need for invasive biopsy.

Dermoscopy: It can be very helpful in diagnosing LS in the extragenital form. The examination can reveal structureless white-to-yellow areas, chrysalis-like structures (suggesting dermal collagen changes), linear irregular blood vessels, keratotic plugs, and perifollicular scaling [24].

Wood's lamp examination: This test uses ultraviolet light to highlight changes in skin pigment. It can be useful in the differential diagnosis to distinguish LS from vitiligo, as it shows fluorescence [23].

Laboratory blood tests

Because lichen sclerosus (LS) is strongly associated with autoimmune diseases, blood tests are often performed to screen for common comorbidities, not to diagnose LS itself. These tests typically include an autoantibody screen, thyroid function tests, complete blood count, and glucose testing (usually as part of a general health screening) [3, 11].

Tests for coexisting conditions

Microbiological: If a secondary infection, such as bacterial or Candida, is suspected to be complicating the LS, swabs for culture can be taken [3].

Patch testing: It may be recommended for patients who respond poorly to treatment or whose biopsy shows features such as eosinophilic spongiosis, which can suggest a superimposed allergic reaction [17].

4. Impact of lichen sclerosus on female sexual function

4.1 Introduction

Lichen sclerosus has a profound and complicated impact, significantly affecting a person's quality of life, mental health, and emotional well-being. The distress is often a direct consequence of the disease's chronic nature, debilitating symptoms, and physical changes [3, 31].

4.2 Mechanism of sexual dysfunction

4.2.1 Physical causes

The pain experienced by patients with lichen sclerosus (LS) is a direct result of physical and anatomical changes to the affected skin.

Thinning of the skin – the skin in LS becomes fragile and thin, making it prone to tearing. Painful cracks, known as fissures, can occur spontaneously or with minor friction, such as during sexual intercourse or defecation. In some cases, the chronic soreness, in combination with the fragility, can lead to erosions, ulcerations, localized haemorrhaging under the skin (purpura or ecchymosis), causing tenderness and pain. Whilst rare, blisters can also form [3, 9].

Scarring (sclerosis) and narrowing – a hallmark of LS, causes the skin to become hardened, inelastic, and whitish-yellow. This scarring can lead to introital stenosis, a narrowing of the vaginal opening. The loss of elasticity and the narrowing make penetration during intercourse difficult and painful (dyspareunia) or even impossible (apareunia) [3, 6, 9].

Atrophy – LS often thins and develops a wrinkled, 'cellophane paper' appearance, making the skin fragile and lacking the normal resilience, which contributes to the risk of fissures and pain during intercourse [3, 32].

Architectural changes and fusion – the chronic inflammation and scarring can lead to significant disfigurement of the vulva, such as fusion or resorption of the labia minora and burying of the clitoris under scar tissue. These architectural changes can cause functional problems and pain, especially during sexual activity [3, 6, 9].

4.2.2 Neurological changes

Lichen Sclerosus (LS) is a debilitating neurological condition characterized by neurogenic inflammation alongside an altered pattern of nerve fibres and nerve receptors in the affected skin.

This study found various changes in the presence of nerve fibre densities depending on the location of the fibre on the skin [32].

- Intraepidermal nerve fibres: The total number of nerve fibres within the epidermis is significantly lower in LS samples compared to healthy skin. This reduction in fibres is indicated to occur as a consequence of the chronic inflammatory autoimmune process [32].

- Subepidermal nerve fibres: Alternatively, the density of nerve fibres located immediately below the epidermis is higher in genital LS than in both extragenital LS and healthy control skin. The apparent increase in subepidermal nerve fibres may help explain why genital LS is the most pruritic form of LS [32].

Calcitonin gene-related peptide (CGRP) is a neuromodulator amine responsible for pain, inflammation, and pruritus. In lichen sclerosus (LS), its expression is significantly altered. The quantity of CGRP-positive nerve fibres is significantly increased in genital LS compared to extragenital LS and healthy controls. This hyperinnervation produced by CGRP-positive fibres is identified in both the intraepidermal layer and the subepidermal layer of genital LS skin. CGRP has vasodilatory and mast cell-activating properties, thereby contributing to neurogenic inflammation. This increased density of CGRP-positive fibres in genital LS can help explain the exaggerated pruritus that is often observed in patients [32].

Vanilloid receptor 1 (VR1), also known as TRPV1, is a receptor that contributes to the transmission of pain and itch sensations. In skin affected by lichen sclerosus (LS) – importantly in both genital and extragenital LS – VR1 is expressed in CGRP-positive fibres, which is abnormal. This coexpression of VR1 and CGRP is not observed in control skin. This indicates a pathological feature of LS and highlights the role that VR1 plays in the pathogenesis of LS, particularly when we consider that VR1 is not normally present in nerve fibres in unaffected skin [32].

These findings have prompted researchers to suggest that neurogenic inflammation is a primary pathogenic mechanism in lichen sclerosus [32].

4.2.3 Hormonal changes

LS research suggests that it is more of an autoimmune disorder than a hormonal disorder. Some association has been found between hyperestrogenism and LS, and lower vulvar androgen receptor expression has been observed in a small population of patients [14]. However, no direct correlation has been established between hormonal changes and LS. Therefore, the current conclusion of the available research is that the postmenopausal changes affecting women, along with the architectural and psychological changes, contribute to sexual dysfunction as a combination rather than hormonal changes alone [33].

4.3 Psychological effects

Living with LS can be emotionally draining. Many women feel distress and anxiety as they navigate their daily lives with a chronic condition that is often misunderstood. The condition negatively impacts self-image, diminishes how women feel about themselves, and reduces their self-esteem [31]. Amongst the many contributing psychological factors, a significant stressor is the increased risk of developing SCC [3]. Studies show that chronic conditions such as LS can lead to anxiety and depression [3]. One study found that two-thirds of those with chronic vulvar disease were diagnosed with a mental health disorder, with mixed anxiety-depressive disorder and depressive episodes being diagnosed most frequently [21]. Notably, the most significant risk factors were the length of the disease and the severity of the itching [21]. The itching can be so severe that sleep is impaired, and women feel such an urge to scratch that it seems unmanageable and embarrassing [9]. This condition can limit social activities due to constraints on the clothing they can wear (anything tight can exacerbate symptoms) or the inability to engage in certain sports or activities, such as horse riding or bicycling, which can be too painful to participate in [9]. LS can have a significant negative impact on sexuality and intimate relationships, which can be a major cause of psychological distress. LS is often misdiagnosed, and delays in reaching a correct diagnosis can extend the suffering of the patient and induce anxiety [34]. The psychological effects of lichen sclerosus represent an important part of the burden of the disease. It affects general happiness, self-perception, and mental stability, all of which highlight the need for a holistic management plan that addresses both physical symptoms and significant emotional and psychological effects. Patients can benefit from support groups and psychological counselling.

4.4 Quality of life limitations

Lichen sclerosus has a significant impact on a person's quality of life by interfering with sexual function and self-esteem, which are essential for maintaining interpersonal relationships. Many affected patients experience persistent itching and pain despite successful treatment, and many are concerned about progression to SCC. The lifetime risk of developing vulval SCC in women with lichen sclerosus is 4% to 5% [3].

4.5 Assessment tools and scoring

Standardized scoring systems help quantify the impact of lichen sclerosus on sexual health. The primary instruments identified are as follows (see **table 6**):

Female Sexual Function Index (FSFI) is a 19-item questionnaire used for women that evaluates six key domains of sexual function: desire, arousal, lubrication, orgasm, satisfaction, and pain. Scores range from 2 to 36, with higher scores indicating better function. A score below 26.55 is generally considered indicative of sexual dysfunction. Patients with LS have consistently scored lower than the normal population [33].

The Vulvar Disease Quality of Life Index (VQLI) is a tool specifically designed to measure the quality of life in patients with vulvar diseases, including vulvar lichen

Tool name	Purpose	Domains assessed
FSFI	Measures sexual function	Desire, arousal, lubrication, orgasm, satisfaction, and pain.
VQLI	Measures impact of vulvar conditions	Symptoms, psychosocial impact, and sexual impact.

Table 6.
Assessment tools for evaluating sexual function in LS.

sclerosus. The scoring assesses the impact of vulvar disease across several key areas of a patient's life, such as symptoms, anxiety, activities of daily living, and sexuality, along with a total overall score. Whilst not used as the primary assessment tool in all of the provided studies, the VQLI is recognized in systematic reviews as one of several instruments used to evaluate the impact of LS on a person's life, alongside tools such as the Female Sexual Distress Scale and the Dermatology Life Quality Index [14, 33].

4.6 Obstacles in patient communication

Despite treatment, many women have reported persistent pain that worsens during coitus. Many affected individuals feel embarrassment and shame, especially regarding changes to the vulva. Patients may feel uncomfortable and insecure about being intimate with a partner and can be reluctant to speak about the disease [3, 34]. This fear can be alleviated with proper information, consistent treatment, and regular follow-ups.

5. Management and therapeutic interventions

5.1 Management overview

The management of LS is a lifelong process involving symptom relief, prevention of irreversible anatomical changes and scarring, and reduction of malignant transformation risk. Since a cure is not yet available, treatment focuses on managing the chronic, relapsing nature of the disease. Management includes topical corticosteroids as first-line therapy, second-line or adjunctive therapies in cases of refractory disease, surgical options for complications, and careful long-term follow-up along with patient education [17, 34, 35].

5.2 Medical management

5.2.1 First-line therapy: corticosteroids

Potent or ultrapotent topical corticosteroids are recognized as the gold-standard and first-line treatment worldwide for all age groups [3].

- Studies show that topical corticosteroids, such as clobetasol propionate 0.05%, provide at least a 75% to 90% improvement in lichen sclerosus (LS) compared to placebos. They are beneficial for reducing inflammation and providing relief from complications such as pruritus and pain. Early and consistent treatment can possibly prevent scarring and most likely reduce the risk of SCC [17, 22, 36, 37].

- A conventional first-line treatment approach involves the application of ointment once daily for up to three months to achieve clinical remission, followed by a tapering regimen and a long-term maintenance plan that may include applying the steroid ointment once or twice a week to keep the disease under control long-term and prevent relapses. Ointments are preferred (over creams or lotions) because they are better tolerated by patients [3, 9, 32].

The treatment protocol that is followed involves applying clobetasol propionate 0.05% ointment once daily at night for 4 weeks, then on alternate nights for 4 weeks, and then twice weekly for further 4 weeks [17].

Extragenital LS can be more resistant to treatment compared to genital LS. Whilst ultrapotent topical corticosteroids are the first-line therapy for genital LS, evidence for their effectiveness on extragenital lesions is more limited. Other therapeutic options include phototherapy (UVA-1 and narrowband UV–B) and systemic treatments such as oral steroids for widespread or refractory cases [18, 21].

5.2.2 Second-line therapy and adjuvants

For patients who are resistant to topical corticosteroids or unable to tolerate them, the options are as follows:

- Topical calcineurin inhibitors – pimecrolimus and tacrolimus – are regarded as second-line agents. They can effectively suppress symptoms such as itching and burning but are generally not as effective as potent steroids in treating the clinical symptoms and inflammation associated with LS [17, 21, 31]. These medications are used off-label, and there is some concern about their long-term safety regarding a potential, though unproven, malignancy risk. Therefore, they are generally not used as a first-line treatment [36].

- Intralesional corticosteroid injections can be an effective substitute for topical treatment when topical agents are ineffective for thick, hyperkeratotic, or resistant lesions [21, 22].

5.2.3 Systemic therapy (methotrexate/retinoids)

For severe, diffuse, or refractory generalized LS, systemic agents can be a last resort and are limited in their use. Retinoids, such as acitretin (dosed at 20–30 mg/day for 16 weeks), can be helpful, but the extent of side effects and teratogenicity limits their use and makes them a specialist option for severe cases that have failed standard therapy [27]. In a small study, topical application of 0.025% tretinoin 5 days a week for 1 year showed good effect [17]. Methotrexate may be used, sometimes in combination with corticosteroids, for refractory generalized extragenital LS [21].

5.3 Surgical management

5.3.1 Indication for surgery

Surgery is not a main stay treatment for LS; it is usually reserved for patients with a high degree of suspicion for malignant transformation and/or for patients with irreversible anatomical scarring [17].

5.3.2 Interventional procedures

Procedures such as perineoplasty, de-adhesion, or synechiolysis may be performed to correct scarring that has led to introital stenosis, which can cause pain during intercourse or problems with urination [21].

5.3.3 Laser and other devices

Phototherapy (UV therapy), especially UVA1, is an effective treatment for extragenital LS. For the treatment of genital LS, it is considered a second-line option due to limited data and concerns about carcinogenicity [17, 18, 21].

Photodynamic therapy is a useful option for vulvar lichen sclerosus (LS) unresponsive to conventional therapy and for symptoms such as pruritus [31].

The use of fractional CO2 laser has been investigated as an adjunct to therapy for vulvar lichen sclerosus (LS) unresponsive to topical steroid therapy, as it has demonstrated some effectiveness in relieving symptoms, improving architectural changes, and enhancing quality of life and sexual function. There is literature that suggests it helps replenish vaginal flora, increase collagenogenesis, promote tissue remodelling, and reverse vaginal atrophy. However, the findings are inconsistent, and therefore, guidelines do not recommend its routine use for LS [38].

5.4 Multidisciplinary management

Supportive care and educating the patient are both important components of managing LS. Emollients and moisturizers are strongly recommended to improve skin barrier function and provide symptomatic relief. Patients should avoid persistent trigger factors such as mechanical friction from tight clothing or specific activities (eg, cycling), scratching, and irritants such as harsh soaps and perfumed products. It is important for patients to understand that LS is a chronic condition, treatment must be adhered to for the long term, and they must be taught how to perform self-examinations to determine if any changes occur (eg, sores, lumps). Additionally, patient support groups should be made available to them [9, 17, 21].

5.5 Special circumstances

5.5.1 Paediatrics

The treatment approach for children is generally more conservative, prioritizing safety and avoiding invasive procedures. The initial treatment with corticosteroids is similar to that for adults; long-term maintenance therapy with low- or mid-potency corticosteroids is typically recommended to continue at least until puberty to prevent scarring and disease progression [17, 21]. The maximum recommended monthly dose of clobetasol propionate for children is approximately 10 grams [26]. Topical calcineurin inhibitors are also suggested as a second-line option or for maintenance therapy. They have been shown to be effective and safe in prepubertal patients; however, the same long-term safety concerns as those for adults apply [27]. There is very little evidence supporting the use of agents such as oral retinoids or methotrexate in paediatric patients, and they are not recommended for routine use. Malignancy risk and follow-up are critical points of divergence. In adults, there is a risk (3–5%) of developing SCC; as such, lifelong follow-up and surveillance are necessary. In prepubertal children, there is no evidence of cancer risk; however, lichen sclerosus (LS) that persists into adulthood carries the same risk as in adults. Therefore, long-term follow-up for children is vital to manage the disease through puberty and into adulthood [26, 38].

5.5.2 Pregnancy

The majority of women with LS showed stable or improved symptoms during pregnancy or experienced varied individual courses of LS. In a prospective study, 45% of pregnant women reported that their LS improved and required less topical corticosteroid therapy, with no cases of worsening symptoms. Other studies report either stable or improved LS outcomes, although approximately half of the women may experience some increase in their symptoms. Rarely, LS may present for the first time during pregnancy. The primary treatment goal is symptom control, with minimal foetal risk [21].

Potent topical corticosteroids are the main treatment during pregnancy. Mometasone furoate is the most recommended for safety reasons, but even more potent agents, such as clobetasol, would be considered safe if used on a small area. Compliance and monitoring postpartum are vital, since there is an increased risk of relapse if topical steroid use decreases following delivery. Continuing treatment is maintained if LS is still present postpartum [21].

Some treatments for lichen sclerosus (LS) are contraindicated in pregnancy, such as topical calcineurin inhibitors and all retinoids, due to the risk to the foetus. Well-controlled LS is not a contraindication for vaginal delivery. LS should not affect perineal wound healing or long-term sexual performance postdelivery. Additionally, antenatal perineal massage is recommended for all pregnant women to reduce the risk of perineal injury [21].

LS can affect men, but it is within the remit of this chapter

5.6 Emerging treatment modalities

Platelet-rich plasma and adipose-derived stem cells have emerged as promising and synergistic treatments for genital lichen sclerosus (LS). They have been shown to significantly improve symptoms such as itching and dyspareunia, reduce the need for corticosteroids, and decrease fibrosis and scarring whilst aiding tissue regeneration. Research is still in its early stages, and more long-term data are needed to establish protocols and long-term efficacy [31].

Biologics such as dupilumab, which work on the IL-4/IL-13 signalling pathway, have been trialled and found to be effective in helping alleviate the hypertrophic symptoms of LS [39].

6. Clinical outcomes and prognosis

6.1 Course of the disease

LS is a lifelong condition requiring ongoing management and surveillance to prevent progression and complications. After initial remission, long-term maintenance therapy with topical corticosteroids (eg, twice weekly) is essential to suppress symptoms, prevent flares, reduce the risk of further scarring, and lower the risk of malignant transformation [9]. Even after successful initial treatment, relapse is common. There have been reports of a relapse rate of 84% at four years [17].

6.2 Response to treatment

Patient adherence to long-term maintenance therapy is a key to preventing relapse and disease progression. One longitudinal study indicated that 93.3% of adherent patients experienced complete disease suppression compared to 35% of partially adherent patients when monitoring disease progression via scarring [17].

6.3 Long-term anatomical outcomes

Lichen sclerosus (LS), especially if it is longstanding or poorly managed, can have a major impact on vulvar architecture in women and girls. Characteristically, it leads to fusion and eventual loss of the labia minora, which is permanent, scarring of the clitoral hood, clitoral phimosis, and narrowing of the vaginal opening, which can result in dyspareunia or difficulty urinating. LS commonly affects the perineum and perianal skin in a characteristic 'figure-of-eight' scar formation, which can lead to inelastic tissue and eventual tearing or bleeding. Without surgical intervention, there is likely to be irreversible vulvar changes. Vulvar scarring is more common in adult women with vulvar LS (79%) compared to girls (20%). The architectural changes to the vulva are irreversible except through surgical intervention, which underscores the importance of early recognition and continual management of LS to control the condition and prevent its progression [17, 26].

6.4 Long-term management

6.4.1 Follow-up protocol

Patients should have regular follow-up examinations with a specialist (dermatologist, gynaecologist, or urologist). The frequency may be every 3–6 months when the disease is active and annually once it has stabilized. These visits are critical for monitoring treatment effectiveness, ensuring adherence, and screening for any signs of SCC [21].

6.4.2 Malignant transformation surveillance

Poor patient compliance with maintenance therapy is a major risk factor for disease progression, scarring, and the development of SCC. One study found that 35% of partially compliant patients experienced progression of scarring, whilst none of the fully adherent patients did [30]. Family surveillance should also be considered, as an increased incidence is seen with anal and genital cancer in individuals with a family history of LS [23, 26].

6.5 Prognosis in special populations

6.5.1 Paediatric

Paediatric LS tends to respond quickly to the use of topical corticosteroids. Studies have shown that 72% of girls become symptom-free, with almost all girls demonstrating considerable improvement when treated with potent or ultrapotent steroids. A three-month course of clobetasol propionate achieved a complete remission rate of 72.6% in girls in one study [26].

6.5.2 Pregnancy

Postpartum is a vulnerable time for possible relapse of LS if treatment is not followed. The risk of relapses from LS has been documented, especially in individuals who have discontinued their TCS treatment, due in part to the physical and emotional demands of caring for a new baby. It is imperative that treatment is continued postpartum if LS is still active [21].

6.5.3 Males

LS can affect men, but it is within the remit of this chapter.

6.6 Psychosocial outcomes

The long-term psychosocial prognosis of LS is influenced by a number of factors. Early diagnosis prevents chronic suffering and irreversible anatomical changes that can impact self-image and sexual function. Maintaining consistent long-term treatment decreases flares, slows progression, and reduces malignancy risk. The best long-term results occur in a multidisciplinary context that treats both physical symptoms and provides psychological care. This should include referrals to pelvic floor physiotherapists, sexologists, and counsellors or support groups to help with the management of functional and emotional aspects of LS. Delayed diagnosis and poor treatment adherence can also contribute to poorer mental health, a lower quality of life, and greater feelings of isolation [3, 21].

6.7 Lifelong monitoring

Monitoring lichen sclerosus over a lifetime is a process created through collaboration between the patient and an established physician. This entails regular clinical evaluations, tracking symptoms and functional impact, and effective patient education on self-examination to help the patient maintain remission, avoid permanent damage, and survey for malignancy.

7. Conclusions

Lichen sclerosus is a chronic inflammatory disease with significant long-term consequences for female sexual health and quality of life. Whilst first-line corticosteroid therapy effectively controls symptoms, relapses are common, and long-term monitoring is required to prevent complications, especially malignant transformation. A multidisciplinary approach combining medical, sometimes surgical, psychological, and rehabilitative strategies is essential for the best outcomes.

Conflict of interest

No conflicts of interest are present for the authors.

Author details

Ramona Ramasamy[1*] and Karishma Hemmady[2]

1 Mersey and East Lancashire Teaching Hospitals, Southend Hospital, Southend-on-Sea, United Kingdom

2 East and North Hertfordshire NHS Trust, Hertford County Hospital, Hertfordshire, United Kingdom

*Address all correspondence to: dr.ramonaramasamy@gmail.com

References

[1] New nomenclature for vulvar disease. New nomenclature for vulvar disease. Journal of Cutaneous Pathology. 1976;**3**(3):159–161. DOI: 10.1111/j.1600-0560.1976.tb01105.x

[2] Baglama Š Š, Jemec GBE, Zmazek J, Trčko K. Sex-related variations in comorbidities in Lichen Sclerosus: A systematic review and meta-analysis. Acta Dermato-venereologica. 2024;**104**(39982). DOI: 10.2340/actadv.v104.39982

[3] Powell J, Wojnarowska F. Lichen sclerosus. Lancet. 2015;**385**(9969): 1777–1789

[4] Baklouti M, Sellami K, Rekik M, Bahloul E, Hammami F, Slim C, et al. Extragenital Lichen Sclerosus: A retrospective study of 17 patients. Indian Journal of Dermatology. 2022;**67**(2):146–149. DOI: 10.4103/ijd.ijd_969_21

[5] De Luca DA, Papara C, Vorobyev A, Staiger H, Bieber K, Thaçi D, et al. Lichen sclerosus: The 2023 update. Frontiers in Medicine. 2023;**10**:1106318. DOI: 10.3389/fmed.2023.1106318

[6] Haefner HK, Aldrich NZ, Dalton VK, Gagné HM, Marcus SB, Patel DA, Berger MB, et al. The impact of vulvar Lichen Sclerosus on sexual dysfunction. Journal of Women's Health. 2014;**23**(9):765–770. DOI: 10.1089/jwh.2014.4805

[7] Jerkovic Gulin S, Lundin F, Eriksson O, Seifert O. Lichen sclerosus—incidence and comorbidity: A nationwide Swedish register study. Journal of Clinical Medicine. 2024;**13**(10):2761. DOI: 10.3390/jcm13102761

[8] Kumari A, Singh PK, Rohatgi R. Vulvar lichen sclerosus: Recent advances in understanding and management. International Journal of Reproduction, Contraception, Obstetrics and Gynecology. 2021;**10**(10):4029–4037. DOI: 10.18203/2320-1770.ijrcog20213887

[9] Kirtschig G. Lichen sclerosus-presentation, diagnosis and management. Deutsches Arzteblatt International. 2016;**113**(19):337–343. DOI: 10.3238/arztebl.2016.0337

[10] Kreuter A, Kryvosheyeva Y, Terras S, Moritz R, Möllenhoff K, Altmeyer P, et al. Association of autoimmune diseases with Lichen Sclerosus in 532 male and female patients. Acta Dermato Venereologica. 2013;**93**(2):238–241. DOI: 10.2340/00015555-1512

[11] Fan R, Leasure AC, Maisha FI, Cohen JM, Little AJ. Thyroid disorders associated with Lichen Sclerosus: A case-control study in the all of us research program. British Journal of Dermatology. 2022;**187**(5):797–799. DOI: 10.1111/bjd.21702

[12] VR A, SK A. Vitiligoid Lichen Sclerosus: A reappraisal. Indian Journal of Dermatology, Venereology, and Leprology. 2008;**74**:118–121

[13] Tran DA, Tan X, Macri CJ, Goldstein AT, Fu SW. Lichen sclerosus: An autoimmunopathogenic and genomic enigma with emerging genetic and immune targets. International Journal of Biological Sciences. 2019;**15**(7):1429–1439. DOI: 10.7150/ijbs.34613

[14] Popa A, Dumitrascu MC, Petca A, RC P, Sandru F. Vulvar lichen sclerosus: Navigating sex hormone dynamics and pioneering personalized treatment paradigm. Journal of Personalized Medicine. 2024;**14**(1):76. DOI: 10.3390/jpm14010076

[15] EG Jr F, Kalra PS. Serum levels of sex hormones in vulvar Lichen Sclerosus, and the effect of topical testosterone. New England Journal of Medicine. 1984;**310**(8):488–491. DOI: 10.1056/NEJM198402233100803

[16] Taylor OA, Birse KD, Hill DJ, Knodel S, Noel-Romas L, Myers A, et al. The relationship between the vaginal and vulvar microbiomes and Lichen Sclerosus symptoms in post-menopausal women. Scientific Reports. 2024;**14**(1):27094. DOI: 10.1038/s41598-024-78372-9

[17] Fistarol SK, Itin PH. Diagnosis and treatment of lichen sclerosus: An update. American Journal of Clinical Dermatology. 2013;**14**(1):27–47. PMID:23329078; PMCID:PMC3691475. DOI: 10.1007/s40257-012-0006-4

[18] Uthayakumar AK, Kravvas G, Bunker CB. Extragenital lichen sclerosus arising in tattooed skin. BMJ Case Reports. 2022;**15**(1):e246216. PMID:34992057; PMCID:PMC8739425. DOI: 10.1136/bcr-2021-246216

[19] Virgili A, Borghi A, Cazzaniga S, Di Landro A, Naldi L, Minghetti S, et al. New insights into potential risk factors and associations in genital Lichen Sclerosus: Data from a multicentre Italian study on 729 consecutive cases. Journal of the European Academy of Dermatology and Venereology. 2017;**31**:699–704

[20] Untaaveesup S, Kantagowit P, Leelakanok N, Chansate P, Eiumtrakul W, Pratchyapruit W, et al. The association between cardiovascular risk factors and Lichen Sclerosus: A systematic review and meta-analysis. Journal of Clinical Medicine. 2024;**13**(16):4668. DOI: 10.3390/jcm13164668

[21] Kirtschig G, Kinberger M, Kreuter A, Simpson R, Günthert A, van Hees C, et al. EuroGuiderm guideline on lichen sclerosus—Treatment of Lichen Sclerosus. Journal of the European Academy of Dermatology and Venereology. 2024;**38**(10):1874–1909. DOI: 10.1111/jdv.20083

[22] Corazza M, Schettini N, Zedde P, Borghi A. Vulvar lichen sclerosus from pathophysiology to therapeutic approaches: Evidence and prospects. Biomedicines. 2021;**9**(8):950. DOI: 10.3390/biomedicines9080950

[23] Wu L, Wang H, Zhang R. Unilateral extragenital lichen sclerosus following Blaschko's lines. Clinical Case Reports. 2024;**12**(12):e9581. DOI: 10.1002/ccr3.9581

[24] Mahajan SA, Dave JS. Dermoscopic evaluation of extragenital Lichen Sclerosus et atrophicus. Dermatology Practical & Conceptual. 2022;**12**(3): e2022125. DOI: 10.5826/dpc.1203a125

[25] Aróstegui Aguilar J, Loidi L, Hiltun I, Larrea M, Cascante L, JI Y. Pediatric genital Lichen Sclerosus: A case series of 11 girls. Anales Del Sistema Sanitario de Navarra. 2022;**45**(3):e1014. DOI: 10.23938/ASSN.1014

[26] Orszulak D, Dulska A, Niziński K, Skowronek K, Bodziony J, Stojko R, et al. Pediatric vulvar Lichen Sclerosus

—a review of the literature. International Journal of Environmental Research & Public Health. 2021;**18**(13):7153. DOI: 10.3390/ijerph18137153

[27] Dinh H, Purcell SM, Chung C, Zaenglein AL. Pediatric Lichen Sclerosus: A review of the literature and management recommendations. The Journal of Clinical and Aesthetic Dermatology. 2016;**9**(9):49–54

[28] Torres A, Zaborek-Łyczba M, Łyczba J, Mertowska P, Mertowski S, Grywalska E. The importance of immunological disorders in the pathogenesis of Lichen Sclerosus in pediatric patients: A systematic review. International Journal of Molecular Sciences. 2022;**23**(22):14212. 14212. DOI: 10.3390/ijms232214212

[29] National Institute for Health and Care Excellence (NICE). Pruritus vulvae. 2022. Available from: https://cks.nice.org.uk/topics/pruritus-vulvae/ [Accessed: 2022-October]

[30] Day T, Selim MA, Allbritton JI, Scurry J. ISSVD Difficult Pathologic Diagnoses Committee (DPDC). Nonsclerotic lichen sclerosus: Definition of a concept and pathologic description. Journal of Lower Genital Tract Disease. 2023;**27**(4):358–364. DOI: 10.1097/LGT.0000000000000760

[31] Paganelli A, Contu L, Condorelli A, Ficarelli E, Motolese A, Paganelli R, et al. Platelet-Rich Plasma (PRP) and Adipose-Derived Stem Cell (ADSC) therapy in the treatment of genital Lichen Sclerosus: A comprehensive review. International Journal of Molecular Sciences. 2023;**24**(22):16107. DOI: 10.3390/ijms242216107

[32] Vuković D, Ogorevc M, Tripković I, Puizina-Ivić N, Saraga-Babić M, Mardešić S. The distribution of innervation and immune cell infiltration is different in genital and extragenital variants of lichen sclerosus. Biomolecules. 2022;**12**(12):1767. DOI: 10.3390/biom12121767

[33] Bettolini L, Maione V, Arisi M, Rovaris S, Romanò C, Tomasi C, et al. The influence of genital Lichen Sclerosus on sexual health and well-being: A tripartite comparative analysis. Journal of Lower Genital Tract Disease. 2025;**29**(1):81–87. DOI: 10.1097/LGT.0000000000000851

[34] Vittrup G, Westmark S, Riis J, Mørup L, Heilesen T, Jensen D, et al. The impact of psychosexual counseling in women with Lichen Sclerosus: A randomized controlled trial. Journal of Lower Genital Tract Disease. 2022;**26**(3):258–264. DOI: 10.1097/LGT.0000000000000669

[35] Halonen P, Heikinheimo O, Hadkhale K, Gissler M, Pukkala E, Jakobsson M. Risk factors for Lichen Sclerosus: A case-control study of 43,000 Finnish women. Journal of Lower Genital Tract Disease. 2024;**28**(2):164–168. DOI: 10.1097/LGT.0000000000000796

[36] Chi CC, Kirtschig G, Baldo M, Brackenbury F, Lewis F, Wojnarowska F. Topical interventions for genital Lichen Sclerosus. The Cochrane Database of Systematic Reviews. 2011;**2011**(12):CD008240. DOI: 10.1002/14651858.CD008240.pub2

[37] Alharbi A, Khobrani A, Noor A, Alghamdi W, Alotaibi A, Alnuhait M, et al. Risk of Lichen Sclerosus and Lichen Planus in patients receiving immune checkpoint inhibitors.

International Journal of Environmental Research & Public Health. 2022;**20**(1):580. DOI: 10.3390/ijerph20010580

[38] Stewart K, Javaid S, Schallen KP, Bartlett S, Carlson NA. Fractional CO2 laser treatment as adjunctive therapy to topical steroids for managing vulvar lichen sclerosus. Lasers in Surgery and Medicine. 2022;**54**(1):138–151. DOI: 10.1002/lsm.23476

[39] Peterson DM, Damsky WE, Vesely MD. Treatment of Lichen Sclerosus and hypertrophic scars with dupilumab. JAAD Case Reports. 2022;**23**:76–78. DOI: 10.1016/j.jdcr.2022.03.002